Praise from Readers

"Scary fact; if your health declines from an inflammatory related disease, you become another number in the medical system and your chance of living an optimal life is slim to none. Who would have known that the cause for so many 2020 pandemic mortalities could have been avoided and that too many people are currently at high risk for subsequent fatal illness if they don't do something about it? How can someone turn this around when the science of optimal health is so incredibly confusing and complex? Dive into The Gut Revolution. Dr Bishara gives clear and concise information with "things to remember" at the end of each chapter to help you take your health back into your own hands and out of the hands of doctors. This is a must read for all."

—Jennifer "JZ" Zerling, MS, CES, CPT
Fitness and Age Management Expert
CEO of JZ Fitness

"Dr. Christine Bishara doesn't just focus on gut health in her day to day practice, she's now also packaged her knowledge up into a neatly organized book. Chapters are easy to get through, and describe the various angles of gut-body connection in simplistic terms that can be easily followed. I recommend this book to anyone who wants an overview of what we know about gut health today. You'll not only love it as a handy resource for yourself, but also to impress friends in conversation on your next meal out."

—Dana Corriel, MD
Board-Certified Internist,
Founder of SoMeDocs, LLC

"This ground breaking book will change your life.

"The Gut Revolution" is a true health-preservation, health promotion "Revolution."

Dr. Bishara simplifies complex scientific principles so that you, the reader, can immediately and easily apply it to your daily life. Her conclusions are startling and based on solid scientific research.

Simply put…this book is a must read!"

—Nabil Fanous, MD, Facial Surgeon,
Best Selling Author and Associate Professor,
McGill University

"Change your gut, change your skin! Dr. Bishara offers revolutionary links between gut dysbiosis and common skin concerns. The innovative solutions prove that a healthy gut is the ultimate secret to radiance from within!"

—Tiffany Moon, MD,
Author of Joy Prescriptions,
Founder of LeadHer Summit

"Dr. Bishara has done what I wish more medical professionals had the courage to do. After listening to her patients as they navigated the unthinkable disruption of a worldwide pandemic, she uncovered big problems that needed to be solved.

Her masterpiece, "The Gut Revolution" happens when a trailblazing student of science enters conversations to achieve results. I've been on the receiving end of Dr. Bishara's care and wisdom and hunger to learn more. She exceeded what I expected as a patient. After you read her unique and brilliant comprehensive, research- rich guide, you'll understand more about your body and be armed as an advocate for its longevity."

—Jeanne M. Stafford
President, Stafford & Company

"*The Gut Revolution explores the vital role gut health plays in overall well-being. Dr. Bishara simplifies complex scientific concepts, making the book accessible to readers of all levels.*

Key highlights include the book's holistic view on gut health, gut bacteria, and lifestyle impacts like diet and stress. Simple and practical strategies are provided by the author to empower readers to enhance their gut health through easy to understand tactics that work.

The chapter on intermittent fasting was especially interesting because it explains how, when done right, the body uses it for immune health and weight loss without severe caloric restriction. This book is a must for anyone wanting to learn more about their body and improve their physical and mental health."

—Françoise Sidime, Ph.D
Founder of Ekarus Global Science

"*The way The Gut Revolution explains the science of your health is like nothing I've ever read. Dr. Bishara is gifted at breaking down ideas and showing you how to heal, but it's more than that. She's a master at explaining the WHY. She gives you a heightened awareness of what's going on in your own body, so you have a mental picture of the changes and the progress you're making. Once you have that, it's easy to stay on track. This book is empowering and transformative.*"

—Claudia Mayer,
Homeopathy student

THE GUT REVOLUTION

Your Roadmap to Lasting Immune Health, Improved Mood, and Weight Control

Christine Bishara, MD

Global Book
Publishing

The Gut Revolution
Christine Bishara, MD
©2024 Christine Bishara, MD. All rights reserved.

ISBN: 978-1-964644-07-3
Book Design & Publishing done by:
Global Book Publishing
www.globalbookpublishing.com
Author headshot by Melanie Wesslock Photography

This book is dedicated to my husband, Jon, and my three children—Lauren, Emma, and Matthew for the countless "draft reviews" they endured. I would also like to acknowledge and thank my extended family members and friends who have also made contributions, reviewed drafts, and given suggestions for this book

Welcome to Your Gut Health Journey!

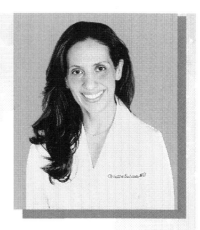

Dr. Christine Bishara is an integrative physician specializing in Internal Medicine. With over **20 years** of experience, she believes in the body's innate healing power but recognizes the need for proper tools and guidance.

She emphasizes the crucial **mind-body connection and advocates for gut health** to enhance overall bodily functions and immune strength.

Dr. Bishara is a pioneer in gut health, having published the first peer-reviewed study linking **COVID-19** severity to a deficiency in beneficial gut bacteria, suggesting this as a reason why children were less severely affected by the virus.

Dr. Bishara discusses the gut and related microbiomes in this book to lead people toward a healthy lifestyle. Understanding the intricate connections between various biological processes and substances is essential for appreciating how our bodies function and maintain health.

To learn more about gut health, scan the QR code and download our free Starter Guide.

Table of Contents

Introduction

I am a big believer that your body is the best doctor, and my hope in writing this book is to provide the reader with the tools and knowledge that took me 30 years to learn. As an obese child and adolescent suffering from eczema, no doctor I saw was able to help me uncover the underlying factors. The traditional 1980's calorie-cutting diets didn't work for me and being bullied for the way I looked in school didn't help my mental health either. It wasn't until the summer of my sophomore year in high school that I took matters into my own hands. That summer, an annual pediatrician well visit was the wake-up call I needed. After my weigh-in for the visit, my doctor emphatically pronounced that I was 60 pounds overweight and that I would never lose the weight. That was my motivation to prove her wrong.

My journey to wellness started that summer when I discovered something interesting about my body. I could still lose weight and not feel deprived if I ate anything I wanted, but mostly nutritious, whole foods, while limiting my eating times. I had inadvertently/instinctively discovered intermittent fasting, although it was not even a thing back then. It worked. I ended up losing 30 pounds that summer.

It wasn't until my first year of medical school, while studying metabolic cycles, that I realized why restricting eating times had been so successful for me. I lost the remaining 30 pounds during medical school by honing in on my body's ability to utilize internal pathways, which not only made me feel better physically, but also had a positive impact on my mental health. I couldn't pinpoint it then, but I discovered something had also changed on a neurochemical level. Now, knowing all I know about the gut **microbiome**, what I felt and continue to feel is not in my imagination, but in fact, due to actual science. Almost every chapter of this book is one that I can relate to personally. I hope that, in the time it takes you to read this book, you will be empowered to understand your body intimately and utilize what took me 30 years to learn.

The chapter on the relationship between COVID-19 and the gut, more specifically, the deficiency of a crucial beneficial gut bacteria, Bifidobacterium, is a discovery I stumbled upon during the pandemic. It is one that, without my love of the gut from a young age, I would probably have overlooked. My discovery was sparked by a spontaneous conversation between myself and my husband, an ICU physician treating patients on the frontline from the start of the pandemic. The published scientific review study on this discovery was the first of its kind to link the gut to COVID-19 severity. Children have much more of this beneficial bacteria, which explains why they don't get very sick from COVID. While there was initial speculation as to how something as simple as a gut bacterial deficiency could cause such a difference, countless other studies have been published since then that point to the same conclusion.

The relationship between the gut and the rest of the body is intricate. Each chapter delves into various aspects of this complexity. Although the chapters may seem disjointed at first, by the conclusion of the book, you will be able to see how all the pieces fit together.

This book will provide you with easy-to-absorb information and tips: easy-to-implement, actionable takeaways, and practical guidance. My hope is to empower you to take charge of your gut health, which translates into improved mental and physical well-being. Use this book as a handy guide while on your health journey.

In health,

Christine Bishara, MD

Email: info@fromwithinmedical.com

Scan to Connect

CHAPTER 1

The Gut Microbiome
A Hidden World Within

In this chapter, we'll start to explore the fascinating world of the gut microbiome and its significant impact on our health—which we will then unlock in greater detail in the following chapters. Scientists are increasingly starting to realize that gut health is critical to overall health and wellness, and we can use this information to revolutionize how we treat our bodies as a whole.

Your gut contains a vast ecosystem of trillions of organisms. Surprisingly, they actively communicate with various parts of the body, including your brain. We're going to explore how these trillions of organisms can impact different aspects of our health, including our mood and possibly even our personalities. These gut **microbes** also maintain connections with our immune system, which is heavily present in the gut and influences how we respond to disease and infections. These organisms are extremely important in determining who we are and how we function from day to day, but few of us even realize that they exist.

The Gut Microbiome

The gut in technical terms consists of the gastrointestinal (GI) tract starting in the mouth, extending to the esophagus, stomach, small and large intestines, and ending at the anal canal. For the purposes of this book, we will focus more on the lower GI tract. These important abdominal organs consist of structures that allow the food you eat to pass through the body. The intestines, although folded neatly in the abdomen, are quite long, measuring 20–25 feet in adults, but that's only the start of it. On a microscopic level, the inner lining of the gut is further folded and compressed, such that the actual surface area of the gut, if completely unfolded, could be as much as 2700 square feet. That's as big as a standard-size tennis court!

The entire surface of the lower GI tract is coated with a thin layer of microorganisms—well over a trillion organisms, including thousands of different species of bacteria, fungi, and viruses. Like any society of organisms, there are beneficial citizens and harmful ones. Beneficial members of the gut ecosystem help to digest the food you eat, process and eliminate toxins, and produce useful byproducts. Their work, however, is always susceptible to disruption by their not-so-beneficial counterparts. Maintaining a healthy balance and harmony among this vast community is crucial. When there is peace and cooperation, the gut and your body function at their best.

Whether you like it or not, whether you know it or not, you are the CEO of this enterprise. The executive decisions you make on a daily basis shape the functioning of the gut. Make healthy choices and you will attract superstar employees who go above and beyond for the company's cause. Neglect your gut and the workplace will soon become overrun by mediocrity and dysfunction.

Like any highly productive workforce, your gut employees need to be fed and since they live inside your gut, what you eat is what they eat. In this book, we'll delve into all the major elements you'll need to boost the beneficial organisms and keep your gut healthy. While I don't like strict dietary restrictions of any kind, the key to a healthy gut lies in adopting a varied diet with an abundance of plant-based, fiber-rich foods that support the growth of beneficial gut strains.

We'll also explore the importance of seemingly small things, like why vitamin D deficiency can significantly impact your gut health or why certain genetic variations can impact your health.

Variation Is Key: Bacterial Diversity and Its Importance

The food you eat plays a role in shaping the diverse population of bacteria in your gut. A varied diet is key to making them happy. Productive and healthy organisms in your gut love to feed on certain foods—mostly plant-based, fiber-rich foods. They love fiber, and the more varied the plant-based fibers, the better. For example, if you eat mangoes, you might be supporting one specific type of beneficial bacteria, while apples or broccoli might support another. This is why it's crucial to emphasize plant-based diversity to support varied beneficial strains of gut microbes.

On the other side of the scale—no pun intended—eating many processed and unhealthy foods can empower harmful gut bacteria, leading to insatiable cravings and an unfavorable balance between good and bad microbes. The more you feed the bad microbes, the more they multiply and the more unhealthy foods they desire. Over time, they'll outnumber and drive out the beneficial microbes you want to encourage. When these harmful microbes start to take over the spaces in the gut lining where beneficial microbes reside, they weaken the lining and start a cascade of leaky gut and inflammation. Maintaining a healthy, balanced, and diverse society of microbes in the gut promotes optimal health.

A study conducted by the Human Microbiome Project found that individuals with higher gut bacterial diversity had better overall health compared to those with lower diversity. High bacterial diversity is associated with improved immunity, reduced inflammation, and protection against various diseases, including type 2 diabetes and **inflammatory bowel disease (IBD)**.

Based on these findings, most experts agree that you should aim to eat 25–30 different plant-based foods like legumes, fruits, and vegetables per week. This will give you the best chance of creating a diverse microbiome that supports a wide range of bacteria. Does this mean you can't have any animal protein? Not necessarily. Later, we'll see how a delicate balance of animal protein can play a role in a healthy diet.

The presence of an imbalance of microbes in the gut is known as **dysbiosis**. Dysbiosis exists when the ratio of beneficial to harmful bacteria begins to reverse. This unhealthy state has been linked to numerous health issues such as:

- **Irritable bowel syndrome (IBS)**
- Inflammatory bowel disease–ulcerative colitis and Crohn's disease (IBD)
- Obesity
- Type 2 diabetes

- Coronary artery disease
- Mental health disorders, such as anxiety and depression

Many factors have been shown to lead to gut dysbiosis:

- **Diet**: A diet high in processed foods, sugar, and unhealthy fats will feed unwanted gut microorganisms, upsetting the balance and pushing out the beneficial bacteria by creating an unsuitable environment for them.
- **Stress**: Chronic stress can lead to inflammatory changes in the gut, also driving out beneficial organisms.
- **Chronic antibiotic use**: While antibiotics are essential for treating bacterial infections, they can also disrupt the balance of good gut bacteria, upsetting the ratios and giving harmful bacteria the opportunity to thrive.
- **Environmental toxins**: Exposure to harmful chemicals in our environment can contribute to dysbiosis by destroying and weakening the gut lining.
- **Alcohol**: Alcohol can deplete the levels of beneficial gut bacteria and weaken the gut lining.

Prebiotics, Probiotics, and Postbiotics: What's the Difference?

You're probably already familiar with these terms, but many people are unsure of the differences, so let's break them down.

Prebiotics are the nondigestible fibers found in various plant-based foods. They serve as the main source of fuel for beneficial gut bacteria. Some of the most nutritious prebiotic-rich foods include:

- Chicory root
- Jerusalem artichoke
- Cruciferous vegetables like broccoli and cauliflower
- Onions
- Garlic
- Asparagus
- Green bananas
- Legumes such as lentils and beans

Consuming a diet rich in prebiotics can help promote bacterial diversity and support overall gut health. Remember, the more variety you consume, the more beneficial microorganisms you will be able to support.

Probiotics are the actual, beneficial live microorganisms. When consumed in adequate amounts, they improve the diversity of gut bacteria. They can be found in fermented foods or probiotic supplements.

Some common probiotic-rich foods include:

- Yogurt
- Kefir
- Sauerkraut
- Kimchi
- Miso
- Tempeh

Incorporating probiotics into your diet can help prevent and alleviate various digestive issues, boost immunity, and improve mental health.

Nourishing a healthy gut goes beyond relying on probiotics as a quick fix. I frequently tell my patients: "You can't probiotic your way out of an unhealthy gut." They are *supplements*; they don't feed the existing microorganisms. You still need to nourish your gut with proper foods, especially prebiotic fibers.

In the world of the "gut workplace," think of prebiotics as the food you give to your company's employees and probiotics as specialists you bring in to enhance their skills. Insufficient levels result in lazy employees who don't perform. Getting enough of both will nurture rockstar employees that get the job done.

Postbiotics are the substances or byproducts that the gut microbes make as they break down the food in your gut. These products are useful in promoting the health of not only the gut but your body as a whole.

A type of postbiotic worth mentioning is a **short-chain fatty acid** (SCFA). SCFAs are produced when gut microbes break down dietary fiber. SCFAs are an important nutrient source for the cells that line your gut. SCFAs help with the digestive process and fortify the integrity of the gut lining. Without these critical substances, the gut lining can become weak and porous, a condition known as leaky gut syndrome. Once the gut barrier is damaged, any toxin or harmful chemical in the gut has an easier time penetrating into your body. Instead of eliminating these toxins in the stool, they now have a port of entry into your bloodstream. This breakdown of your body's defenses has been associated with increased gut inflammation, reduced immune function, poor absorption of key nutrients like calcium and magnesium, and even increased risk of colon cancer.

Some important SCFAs are butyrate, propionate, and acetate, which we will discuss in later chapters. Other postbiotics include **neurotransmitters**, certain enzymes, and vitamins.

Feeling full? Postbiotic butyrate can influence signaling pathways in the brain and the satiety center.

Other Important Factors Affecting the Gut

Vitamin D Deficiency

The continent of Africa has the lowest incidence of colon cancer in the world. Could sunshine play an important role? Abundant sunshine and a much lower incidence of vitamin D deficiency than in other parts of the world may give us clues.

Traditional African diets are also abundant in fiber-rich root-based foods. These are often complemented by ample sun exposure, providing a natural source of vitamin D. The importance of vitamin D extends beyond its role in maintaining strong bones; it also acts as a crucial cofactor in the gut, contributing to the regulation of the immune system. It is important to note that Africa also has a low incidence of IBD compared to industrialized nations such as the United States and Europe. Could the combination of vitamin D, a high-fiber diet, and low consumption of processed foods be protective of our gut microbiome?

Research indicates that individuals diagnosed with colon cancer also frequently suffer from vitamin D deficiencies, which suggests a potential link between the deficiency and this particular type of cancer.

Vitamin D has a protective effect, working in tandem with specific gut bacteria to regulate important mediators released by our immune system. Notably, the connection between vitamin D and gut health was further highlighted during the COVID-19 pandemic, where individuals with vitamin D deficiencies showed reduced recovery rates, underscoring the importance of the gut's influence on overall health. More interestingly, vitamin D helps support some of our beneficial gut bacteria, such as Bifidobacteria.

Boosting Your Vitamin D

My wellness checks always include a vitamin D screen with bloodwork. Eight out of 10 of my patients have levels below the normal range and the ones within the "reference range of normal" (20 ng/mL) are still not enough by my standard. In my opinion, your levels need to be between 40 and 80 ng/mL to be considered optimal. You can increase your vitamin D levels by getting 15–20 minutes of sunshine daily. I also frequently recommend vitamin D supplementation.

Things to Remember

- **It's all about the microbiome:** The gut microbiome plays a crucial role in overall health. Maintaining bacterial diversity is essential for optimal well-being.
- **Dysbiosis has consequences:** An imbalance in the gut microbiome can lead to various health issues, including digestive disorders, obesity, and mental health problems.
- **You need all the biotics:** Incorporate a wide variety of prebiotic and probiotic-rich foods into your diet to support a healthy gut microbiome.
- **Ask your doctor:** Before making any major dietary changes, consult with a healthcare professional or nutritionist to create a personalized plan for improving gut health.
- **Make small daily changes:** Minimize stress, limit exposure to environmental toxins, and avoid unnecessary antibiotic use to help maintain a balanced gut microbiome.

CHAPTER 2

Your Gut

The Immune System Command Center

The gut microbiome and your immune system are intricately linked. As we have explored in Chapter 1, the gut takes up a large surface area in your body. Everything you eat and drink passes through the gut, thus maintaining the health of this barrier is crucial.

Meet Your Immune System

The immune system is an extraordinary network of both cells and messengers. These cells and messengers work together to fight dangerous invaders and substances. The human immune system is quite complex and although it is present in every part of the body, it is estimated that approximately 70% of the immune system is housed within the gut. It would require an entire book to fully understand the immune system, but in simpler terms, the cells of the immune system all have different functions such as attacking foreign or toxic substances, or recording information about previously encountered invaders in the event of a future exposure. The messaging portion of the immune system sets up a communication network that coordinates signals between these components.

Our immune system is always ready to step in when it senses an intruder. Some important immune cells are **T cells** and **B cells**.

T cells are types of white blood cells. These are some of the types:

- *Cytotoxic T cells*: Directly kill foreign cells.
- *Helper T cells*: These call on other immune system cells to help fight foreign invaders.
- *Memory T cells*: These remember previous invaders and help your body react to them quickly the next time around.

B cells are also types of white blood cells. They make antibodies, which are large proteins that, when encountering a dangerous or foreign substance, can attach to it, either killing it or sounding the alarm to the rest of the immune system. Since these substances are freely floating at all times in the immune system, their response to invasion can be immediate.

T and B Cells: The Body's Scorekeepers

The popular phrase "an elephant never forgets" is due to the fact that elephants have superb memories. The human immune system also has a superb memory. It activates T memory cells to take note of what the body encounters and remembers it. The body's defenses are partly dependent upon T memory cells. Once a T memory cell learns something, it rarely forgets it. This is partly how natural immunity develops.

When these cells encounter a virus or harmful bacteria for the first time, they respond by taking offensive action, but they don't always get it right initially. When these cells encounter a virus for the second time, they can recall the previous encounter and know how to mount a proper response to it. The response will become more efficient each time. Your immune system learns to become more effective by expanding its database as you encounter more diseases. Unfortunately, viruses and bacteria are also smart and can make slight changes in their configuration to trick our immune systems into thinking they haven't encountered them before. The healthier and more robust the immune system, the faster and more effectively it will be able to deal with the infection, and this is partly reliant on T memory cells, along with B cells that make antibodies.

The Immune System You're Born with versus the Immune System You Develop

Your **innate immune system** is what you're born with. It is your body's first line of defense against any intruders, and it responds to anything it doesn't recognize, but in a nonspecific way. Since it doesn't yet recognize individual diseases, it will fight anything unfamiliar and try to drive it out of the body.

Your adaptive immunity is the immunity you develop over time, which also works to protect you—but it's slower and more specific. Your adaptive immunity is the part that keeps a database of diseases, figures out how to handle them, and creates a specific, targeted defense against invaders. It will recognize particular pathogens and establish records of how to deal with them.

Your gut microbiome supports both of these systems. It helps to modulate your immune responses, allowing your body to produce inflammation when necessary.

The Role of Short-Chain Fatty Acids in Modulating Immune Responses

Short-chain fatty acids (SCFAs) have been mentioned in Chapter 1, but we haven't yet looked at their amazing role in modulating your immune responses. SCFAs like acetate, butyrate, and propionate are produced when your gut bacteria ferment dietary fiber, and they're a crucial part of the immune system's functioning.

Firstly, SCFAs help to regulate T cell functioning. SCFAs can turn on various kinds of responses, affecting how certain messengers behave in inflammatory responses. A sufficient number of SCFAs ensures that these messengers behave as they should and maximizes the chances of the body producing a valid immune response.

SCFAs help your body properly regulate its immune response once a threat has been dealt with, which lowers the level of inflammation in your body and may help to prevent long-term inflammation and the associated problems that this causes.

What Happens When Our Immune System Is Always on the Frontlines?

A common problem that can occur with our immune system is when it's always "on alert." This leads to inflammation signals always being active, causing chronic inflammation. A big culprit of chronic inflammation is gut dysbiosis. Lazy, destructive employees don't protect the gut lining the way beneficial ones do. They don't produce the postbiotic substances you need; instead, they release toxins and allow some of these toxins to escape into the bloodstream. Additionally, if your immune system isn't working as well as it should because it has become fatigued from the chronic inflammation, it's more likely to misidentify a threat and attack it, and possibly attack the body too. Remember, the immune system is programmed to attack things it doesn't recognize, usually invaders that are threatening the body.

It Starts Early: The Importance of the Gut in Early Childhood

Studies have shown that the first inhabitants in a baby's gut actually come from bacteria in the mother's womb. Intrauterine bacteria pass through the amniotic fluid and then eventually make their way into the gut of a growing fetus. One such bacteria that plays an important role in immune function is a beneficial one called Bifidobacterium (remember that name; it will play a HUGE role in coming chapters, especially when it comes to COVID-19).

Things to Remember

- **Bifidobacterium is essential for the development** of the immune system in early childhood. Maintaining adequate levels is crucial for continued immune health.
- **Leaky gut** is a condition that allows toxins to leak out of our gut and into the bloodstream. This can predispose us to many health issues.
- **SCFAs, produced by gut bacteria,** help regulate immune responses. **Eating foods like** sweet potatoes, peas, lentils, whole grains, and many other plant-based foods will provide our body with nutrients that feed our gut microbes.

CHAPTER 3

What Happened with COVID-19?
The Gut–COVID Connection

COVID-19 provided a glimpse into how our immune systems reacted differently in different individuals.

Gut Bacteria: A Pivotal Role in Immune Function

As we have learned, when substances enter the bloodstream, the immune system must decide whether these substances are safe or unsafe. Remember that the immune system's army is at the frontlines of the body, responding to anything foreign that may enter. These cells and messengers work together to respond in the best way possible. This response can vary, and the immune system may often need to call in more troops or fighters.

Your Immune System's Messengers

Some messengers of the immune system's army are called **interleukins**. So far, research has identified 33 of them, but there may be more. Subsets of these interleukins are called **cytokines** and they also act as important messengers of the immune system.

Cytokines affect how the body responds to intrusions and help with proper signaling when a major immune response occurs.

Interleukins respond to intruders in one of two ways: they can be either pro-inflammatory or anti-inflammatory. It is important that the body releases pro-inflammatory substances, as long as the inflammation is short term. Short-term inflammation helps the body get its "fighters" lined up to deal with whatever it perceives as an impending attack. It also ramps up all the white blood cells and gears your body for the ensuing "battle." The immune system also releases many anti-inflammatory interleukins such as interleukin-10 that prevent excessive inflammation and promote tissue repair. This delicate interplay between pro and anti-inflammatory responders allows these fighters to work together during an "invasion."

One of the pro-inflammatory markers that play an important role in COVID-19 infections is interleukin-6 (IL-6). It is released to rev up the body for attack by creating an inflammatory immune response. Remember, in small doses, inflammation can be helpful. However, if it's released over a prolonged period, it creates a chronic inflammatory state that can cause a range of health issues.

In certain conditions where the body feels the need to be in constant "fight mode," IL-6 levels remain elevated, keeping the body in prolonged "high alert." Persistently elevated IL-6 levels are thought to be a cause of many chronic illnesses and cancers, and can have an effect on how your body responds to illnesses such as COVID-19. In fact, high IL-6 levels were one of the main markers present in those who developed more severe COVID-19 infections.

Why Was the Gut So Important in COVID-19?

Your gut bacteria play a vital role in regulating which interleukins are released and in what quantities. Without them, your body can't regulate a healthy inflammatory response and inflammation can get out of control quickly.

Bifidobacteria is the ultimate beneficial bacteria when it comes to understanding the impacts of COVID-19 on different individuals.

This bacteria is also an especially important microbe when it comes to understanding why COVID-19 has a different impact on children. Bifidobacterium has been identified as being present in very high concentrations in children's guts, comprising up to 60–80% of their gut bacterial composition. Bifidobacterium plays a crucial role in regulating inflammatory pathways within the body. It has been shown to downregulate IL-6, thus reducing chronic inflammation. It also upregulates anti-inflammatory markers such as interleukin-10, further reducing inflammation. It therefore plays an integral role in maintaining the balance within the system. It is what protected children from more severe COVID-19 infections during the pandemic.

While researching COVID-19, my colleagues and I discovered that many of the people who developed severe symptoms had particularly high levels of IL-6. This indicated that their inflammation levels were high—likely chronically high and difficult to control, increasing their susceptibility to severe COVID-19 infections. Many of these same individuals also had risk factors that decreased their Bifidobacterium levels. This was not a coincidence.

Two factors that decrease the levels of Bifidobacterium are advancing age and poor diet. Older adults, individuals who are overweight or obese and those with inflammatory issues such as diabetes and heart disease, tend to have lower levels or even a complete lack of Bifidobacterium. That makes it harder for their bodies to properly regulate the pro-inflammatory effects of IL-6. They end up with chronic unopposed inflammation, which has a detrimental effect on their overall health.

We know that COVID-19 increases inflammation. When a person with chronic inflammation is infected with this virus, the body goes into inflammation overdrive. They cannot regulate the inflammation, which gets out of control and damages important organs and tissues. This is an example of when interleukins such as cytokines flood the body with inflammation to the point that it can't regulate it. The term Cytokine Storm was mentioned frequently when describing individuals who were hospitalized with severe infections and it also explains why some groups were more vulnerable to severe illness from COVID-19.

COVID-19 and the Immune System Response

What actually happens with the immune system when a virus like COVID-19 comes in? The answer depends heavily on the immune system in question. Each immune system is unique and works in a slightly different way.

As discussed, a child's gut contains a large amount of Bifidobacteria. This is nature's way of fortifying their innate immune system as they work on building their **adaptive immune system**. This makes a child's immune regulation different from an adult's. This is why we saw that children often had milder symptoms of COVID-19. Their high levels of Bifidobacterium prevented the IL-6 inflammatory overdrive, which caused the more severe damage seen in some adults. When they were infected with COVID-19, their Bifidobacterium kicked into action quickly to downregulate the inflammation before it got out of hand.

Bacterial concentrations change and generally decrease with time, meaning that your resistance decreases as you age. Adults who have adequate levels of Bifidobacterium in their guts (and while it may not be 60–80%) were also able to regulate the inflammatory overdrive and had milder symptoms. Elderly adults, those with comorbid conditions, such as diabetes and heart disease, or those who are overweight, tend to have low Bifidobacterium levels, some less than 1%. This isn't enough to properly regulate the inflammatory response, which puts the body under immense stress.

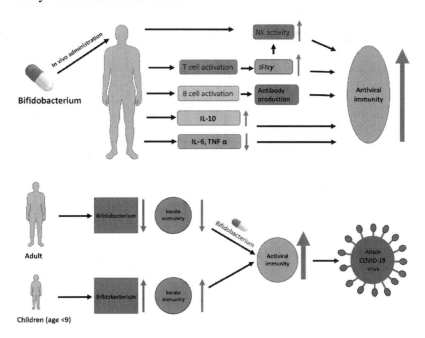

So why do some adults have such low levels? A lot of it comes down to diet and the food we eat. Remember, we aren't just eating for one; we are feeding the numerous organisms in our gut. In many cases, we simply aren't eating well enough to support the beneficial bacterial strains such as Bifidobacterium that help to regulate our immune system.

Gut–Immune Imbalance: The Consequences

When the gut microbiome is imbalanced, it leads to a wide range of problems such as a weakened immune system, making you more susceptible to infections and various health issues. When you don't feed the beneficial gut microbes that help regulate your inflammatory responses, you are more likely to encounter:

- Frequent colds and flu
- Allergies and asthma
- Autoimmune diseases, such as rheumatoid arthritis and multiple sclerosis

Contributing Factors to Gut–Immune Imbalance

The four major factors that affect your immune health are:
- **Diet**: A diet lacking in prebiotic and probiotic-rich foods can negatively impact gut health and immune function.
- **Stress**: Chronic stress can disrupt the balance of gut bacteria and weaken the immune system. Stress also elevates the production of IL-6 and Cortisol,

increasing your body's chance of staying in a chronic inflammatory state.

- **Antibiotic use**: Overuse or nonessential use of antibiotics can kill harmful bacteria, but also beneficial bacteria, leading to a weakened immune response.
- **Environmental toxins**: Exposure to harmful chemicals contributes to an imbalance in gut bacteria. Phthalates and other environmental toxins can increase IL-6, leading to more inflammation within the body and putting more stress on your immune system.

Environmental toxins may be unavoidable, but diet and stress can be managed. A healthy approach to living and a good understanding of prebiotics, probiotics, and fermented foods can improve gut health and immune function.

Very early in the pandemic, I recommended probiotic foods and high-dose probiotic supplements to my patients infected with COVID-19. Vitamin D and zinc were also given during the acute phase. I lost NO ONE with this protocol.

Remember how your T memory cells have great memories? They also played a role in COVID-19. You may recall that there were some news stories about people who had encountered SARS-1 in the past, and then had milder symptoms when they encountered COVID-19 (SARS-2). This may have occurred because their memory cells recalled how to respond to that type of infection. Their bodies were able to respond more effectively because they already had an action plan in their database that told them what to do.

Interesting Facts about Bifidobacterium

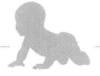

Children have much higher levels in their guts.

Children under the age of 10 have up to 60–80% of their gut occupied by this bacteria. The levels slowly start to decline as we age.

The high levels of Bifidobacterium are nature's way of protecting children while they build a more robust immune system.

Factors That Impact the Levels of Bifidobacterium in Humans

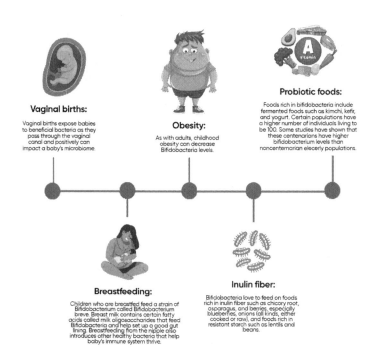

Vaginal births:

Vaginal births expose babies to beneficial bacteria as they pass through the vaginal canal and positively can impact a baby's microbiome.

Obesity:

As with adults, childhood obesity can decrease Bifidobacteria levels.

Probiotic foods:

Foods rich in bifidobacteria include fermented foods such as kimchi, kefir, and yogurt. Certain populations have a higher number of individuals living to be 100. Some studies have shown that these centenarians have higher bifidobacterium levels than noncentenarian elecerly populations.

Breastfeeding:

Children who are breastfed feed a strain of Bifidobacterium called Bifidobacterium breve. Breast milk contains certain fatty acids called milk oligosaccharides that feed Bifidobacteria and help set up a good gut lining. Breastfeeding from the nipple also introduces other healthy bacteria that help baby's immune system thrive.

Inulin fiber:

Bifidobacteria love to feed on foods rich in inulin fiber such as chicory root, asparagus, and berries, especially blueberries, onions (all kinds, either cooked or raw), and foods rich in resistant starch such as lentils and beans.

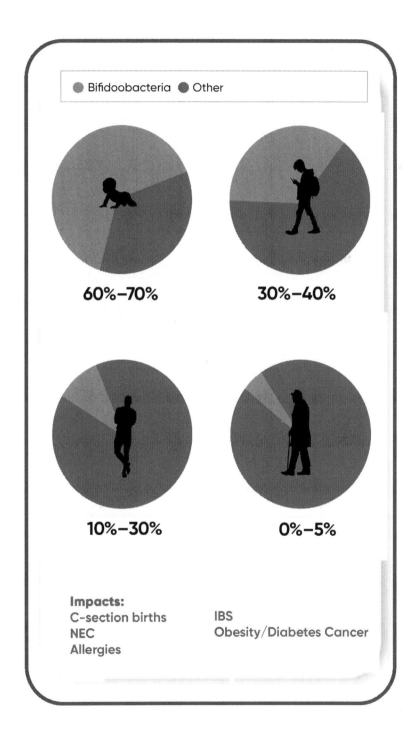

Things to Remember

- **Gut–immune health:** The gut plays a vital role in immune function, with vital beneficial bacteria like Bifidobacterium tremendously impacting our immune system.

- **Gut–immune imbalance consequences:** An imbalance in the gut microbiome can weaken the immune system, causing chronic inflammation, which can lead to the development of chronic illnesses and the inability to handle infections such as COVID-19.

- **The gut–COVID connection:** What we saw during the pandemic was that certain individuals responded differently to COVID, but the majority of children had mild infections and this can be attributed to the fact that Bifidobacterium downregulates the same inflammatory pathways of the immune system that COVID affects. Children have enough bifidobacteria to immediately act and lower the inflammation caused by COVID.

Those with deficient or absent bifidobacteria were not able to control the ensuing inflammation overdrive caused by the Cytokine Storm that caused damage to the body.

- **Diet and lifestyle matter:** Consume a diverse range of plant-based foods, find strategies to manage stress, exercise regularly, and get adequate sleep at night to improve your gut health and immune function.
- **Probiotics and prebiotics are essential:** Incorporate probiotic and prebiotic-rich foods into your daily routine to support a balanced gut microbiome and a healthy immune system.

CHAPTER 4

The Gut's Role

In Autoimmune Diseases and Cancer

Autoimmune diseases and the incidence of cancer have increased dramatically in the past 30 years. It is estimated that the occurrence of both conditions will continue to rise.

The Leaky Gut–Autoimmune Connection

An autoimmune disease is essentially what the name suggests: the immune system releases antibodies to "fight the intruder," except in this case, it's your own body.

Remember, the immune system is programmed to attack things it doesn't recognize, usually invaders that are threatening the body. In autoimmune conditions, the response may be triggered by external substances, and in an attempt to attack these foreign invaders, the body attacks its own cells.

A potential explanation is that our guts are being exposed to a lot of harmful substances and toxins, whether they are leaching out of plastics, coming in with processed foods, or entering from the environment through our skin, etc. The body then stays in inflammation "overdrive" and continues to attack its own cells.

The gut lining is kept strong by short-chain fatty acids (SCFAs). The fatty acids function as "soldiers on the front lines" of the gut lining wall, preventing harmful bacteria from occupying these spaces and keeping toxins out of your bloodstream. The more SCFAs we produce, the stronger the gut lining is in preventing toxic substances from leaking into the bloodstream.

Chronic Inflammation, Meet Leaky Gut; Leaky Gut, Meet Chronic Disease

A leaky gut is a condition that relates to the permeability of the gut lining. Our guts are semi-permeable, meaning they allow water and nutrients to pass from the intestines into the bloodstream. However, some people have increased permeability, which means that other molecules can also pass through, allowing toxins and other harmful substances into the bloodstream, rather than keeping them trapped in the GI tract.

Leaky gut is thought to be a contributing factor in many chronic inflammatory states, illnesses, and autoimmune diseases because it allows harmful molecules to pass into the bloodstream, triggering your body's alarm response. SCFAs, which, as you may recall, are produced by beneficial bacteria in the gut. The fatty acids function as "soldiers on the front lines" of the gut lining wall, preventing bad bacteria from occupying these spaces and keeping toxins out of your blood.

The Gut–Inflammatory Bowel Disease (IBD) Connection

IBD comprises two autoimmune conditions called ulcerative colitis and Crohn's disease. Both cause inflammation in the gastrointestinal (GI) tract. While ulcerative colitis typically affects only the mucosa, the innermost layer of the colon, Crohn's disease can affect any part of the gastrointestinal tract and its inflammation often penetrates multiple layers of the intestinal lining. Both frequently cause other symptoms outside the GI Tract. Peak incidence of diagnosis is during adolescence and young adulthood.

While the treatment for IBD usually involves the regular use of anti-inflammatory and strong immune-modulating medications, many patients have reported improvement in their symptoms from a diet called the *specific carbohydrate diet* (SCD). This diet was created in the 1950s by a physician named Dr. Sidney Haas, who had spent a large portion of his medical career developing a nutritional plan for those suffering from severe IBD. Despite the protocol being present in many scientific and nutritional textbooks, it remained largely unknown. It wasn't until he met Elaine Gottschall, a mom with a very ill 8-year-old daughter with ulcerative colitis. Elaine was told by all doctors that her daughter's only chance of survival was to surgically remove part of her colon. Just before the surgery, a friend of Elaine introduced her to Dr. Haas, and with his help, she put her daughter on his dietary protocol. Her daughter's ulcerative colitis started to heal and she went into remission, never requiring surgery. Her daughter is now in her 70s and still follows the diet. Unfortunately, some 80 years later, this diet is barely known, but I have personally seen many of my patients completely resolve or, at the minimum, improve their IBD symptoms using this approach. Elaine Gottschall wrote a book about this protocol called *Breaking the Vicious Cycle*.

The approach eliminates specific carbohydrate-rich foods, but not all of them. It involves eating nutritious whole foods while eliminating processed foods, sugar, and refined carbohydrates such as breads and pastas. It incorporates certain fiber-rich plant-based foods, but not all of them.

This diet not only works for many with IBD, IBS, and gluten sensitivity, but anyone with an autoimmune disease, chronic medical condition, or gut issues can still benefit from this protocol.

Here is a quick list of the foods allowed on the SCD that have helped many of my patients, as well as others who have educated themselves on a diet's link to gut health.

The Specific Carbohydrate Diet

1. **Foods allowed on the SCD:**
   - Organic meats without additives, including poultry, wild-caught fish, wild shellfish, and organic eggs.
   - Broth from organic chicken or grass-fed beef. This is especially good during flares as the broth is rich in collagen and nutrients that can help heal the gut lining, while limiting the large digestive demand on the gut as it heals.
   - Dairy, limited to hard cheeses such as cheddar, gouda, etc., in small quantities.
   - Homemade yogurt fermented for at least 24 hours, or organic plain yogurt with no added sugar, such as Greek yogurt. Organic kefir is also allowed.

- Most fresh, frozen, raw, or cooked vegetables and string beans.
- Fresh, raw, cooked, frozen, or dried fruits with NO added sugar.
- Most nuts and nut flours.
- Most oils, teas, coffee, mustard, and juices with no additives or sugars.
- Organic honey as a sweetener; Manuka honey is also great.

2. **Prohibited foods on the SCD:**

- Sugar, molasses, maple syrup, sucrose, processed fructose, including high-fructose corn syrup, or any processed sugar.
- All grains, including corn, wheat, wheat germ, barley, oats, rice, and others, as well as bread, pasta, and baked goods made with grain-based flour.
- Canned vegetables with added ingredients.
- Some legumes, such as garbanzo or pinto beans. No canned beans of any kind.
- Seaweed and seaweed byproducts.
- Starchy tubers such as potatoes, sweet potatoes, and turnips.
- Canned and most processed meats.
- Canola oil and commercial mayonnaise due to the additives they contain.
- All milk and milk products that are high in lactose, such as mild cheddar, soft cheeses, commercial yogurt, cream, sour cream, and ice cream.
- Candy, chocolate, and products that contain fructooligosaccharides.

Why This Diet Works: Breaking the Cycle

- *Bacterial overgrowth*: Since they have little fiber, refined carbohydrate-rich foods remain in the intestine longer. These carbohydrates become energy sources for harmful bacteria, leading to bacterial overgrowth. These bacteria release harmful toxins, also known as lipopolysaccharides, which cause injury to the intestinal lining.
- In response to harmful substances, the intestine secretes mucus to create a protective barrier. Unfortunately, this barrier also inhibits digestive enzymes from fully breaking down undigested carbohydrates, resulting in increased bacterial overgrowth and the release of more toxins.
- The inflammation caused by these processes hinders the intestine's ability to absorb nutrients effectively, resulting in malabsorption and malnutrition.
- With all the chaos going on in the intestine, the immune system is triggered to release inflammatory responders, which brings on more inflammation and further damage to the intestinal lining.

If you're suffering from gut issues, it might be worth discussing this diet with your doctor. It helps many individuals with gut health issues, not just those with IBD, because it removes many of the culprits that cause gut inflammation and leaky gut.

Strategies for Preventing and Managing Autoimmune Conditions

It is much better to work on preventing an autoimmune disease rather than treating it. Keeping those gatekeepers alert so that they don't allow intruders or lazy employees means we have to feed them properly and allow them to get rest. The only way to kick the lazy employees out is to attract good employees who get more bang for their buck food-wise and encourage more alert gatekeepers to join the company.

The Cancer Connection: The Gut Microbiome's Influence on Cancer Development

Colon cancer is the deadliest form of cancer for men and the second deadliest cancer for women. There are many risk factors for colon cancer, but improved gut health is a preventable factor that can be easy to implement. The presence of certain strains of microbes can encourage cancer development, while other kinds may be able to suppress the growth of tumors.

For example, high levels of certain strains of bacteria, like Fusobacterium nucleatum, have been linked to colorectal cancer. Fusobacteria are a natural part of the mouth flora, so it's not necessarily about completely eliminating certain kinds of bacteria; it's about maintaining balance. Poor oral hygiene however can allow these organisms to get out of control and increase inflammation, otherwise known as plaque. The same thing can actually happen in the gut when these bacteria form colonies called "**biofilm**." Biofilm is the equivalent of plaque in the mouth, but it is present in the lower GI tract.

While brushing your teeth can decrease much of the plaque in your mouth, there aren't any effective ways to brush your gut. Eating cruciferous vegetables like broccoli, cauliflower, and raw vegetables can act as natural toothbrushes for your gut. The motion of their passing through the gut can help to break down some of the biofilm.

Fusobacteria have also been linked to higher resistance to chemotherapy and increased risk of tumor recurrence. Let's compare that with the effects of beneficial organisms like Bifidobacterium and Lactobacillus. Both of these bacteria can suppress the growth of tumors and could reduce your risk of cancer development, because they release antitumor markers that help destroy cancerous cells. They are capable of taking out cancer cells, but only if they're being supported in the right environment.

Of course, diet isn't all that matters when it comes to cancer, but the gut can play a role in hormone imbalances too, potentially impacting reproductive system cancers as well as breast cancers. Estrogen production is made through different pathways, some of which are healthy, and some of which are not so healthy. If you're not eating the foods that support your beneficial gut bacteria, your body will start utilizing and producing estrogen through unhealthy pathways.

There are three forms of estrogen: estriol, estrone, and estradiol. There is a common saying about estrogen that it has been dubbed both the angel of life and the angel of death. A lot of this depends on which pathway estrogen is produced through. Extensive research has been done by Dr. David Zava, an estrogen expert. He and his team have found that estrogen metabolized down a pathway called the 2-Hydroxy pathway was safer than estrogen metabolized down the 4-Hydroxy pathway, which was found in patients with breast cancer. Healthy estrogen production through the 2-Hydroxy pathway can be influenced by the beneficial organisms in the gut.

A perfect example of an unhealthy type of estrogen is estrone. Fat cells can be converted into this type of estrogen when they are in excess, and estrone is metabolized through the unhealthy "estrogen pathway." Estrogen dominance can increase a person's risk of breast cancer. This is why being overweight, especially after menopause, increases a woman's risk of endometrial, ovarian, and breast cancer.

Vitamin D and Cancer

We've spoken in previous chapters about the important role vitamin D plays in strengthening the gut barrier, so it's a friend of the gatekeepers, so to speak. Certain gut bacteria, in turn, are needed to convert inactive vitamin D into its active form to allow your body to better utilize it.

We've also highlighted the low colon cancer and IBD rates in Africa as clues to help us understand the importance of diet and vitamin D deficiency.

While we don't understand the exact mechanism yet, we do know that vitamin D can also help the immune system figure out how to respond to cancerous cells.

While getting it from the sun is ideal, supplementation is also a reliable way to increase levels. This is probably because daily supplementation is a more consistent method of obtaining vitamin D regularly, and not that the sun is a suboptimal way of absorbing vitamin D. Vitamin D3 is currently thought to be better than vitamin D2. Remember to consult with a doctor before you start taking any form of supplementation because, in rare cases, you can have too much vitamin D.

Things to Remember

- **A leaky gut** could contribute to the development of autoimmune diseases.
- **The gut microbiota** could play a role in the development of autoimmune diseases and cancer, which shows how crucial it is to have a balanced and diverse gut microbiota.
- **The specific carbohydrate diet** has been shown to help heal the gut in patients with IBD or other gut health issues.
- **Colon cancer** is on the rise and diet and vitamin D may play bigger roles in prevention than previously thought.
- **Lifestyle factors,** including diet, physical activity, and stress management, significantly impact gut health and disease risk.
- **Vitamin D** plays a crucial role in gut and immune health, so ensuring adequate intake is essential.

CHAPTER 5

Intermittent Fasting and Gut Health
The Body's Ultimate Spring Cleaning

Fasting has gained a lot of attention in recent years with some incredible health benefits coming from not only WHAT you eat, but also WHEN you eat.

Understanding Fasting: An Ancient Practice with Modern Benefits

While you might only have started to hear about fasting in recent years, it has existed throughout most of human history and our ancestors used it extensively. Fasting is the body's survival mechanism, and it's reflective of the way humans have evolved. In the past, humans didn't have access to food 24/7. They were busy hunting, gathering, and preparing food. They didn't have access to the nearest grocery store to buy anything they desired. This is precisely why our bodies are equipped to survive when we don't have a constant supply of food. The human body actually thrives on these backup survival mechanisms that fuel your cells, so they continue to function. In reality, cells perform better when we eat during these timed windows.

Many people confuse fasting with strict caloric restriction or going days without eating, which is not at all what it means. It may help to view intermittent fasting in terms of "intermittent eating" to better understand the concept.

Fasting doesn't mean starving yourself or going days without food. Instead, it often means eating an adequate amount (or moderate restriction of food if the goal is weight loss) during certain hours of the day. For example, if you're following a Mediterranean-style diet, you can consume mostly plant-based food choices while not restricting any type of food, but instead, eating within a specific time window. When done in a sensible manner, my motto is "Eat whatever you want, but not whenever you want."

My Personal Fasting Journey

As an obese teen, my impetus for change came the summer of my sophomore year of high school. My mom, sister, and I had gone on a cruise to Bermuda. As is the protocol on these ships, the Captain's Dance Night was one of the highlighted events. Just as the dance started, a stranger approached my mom and older sister to dance, but they politely declined. He took a look at me and walked away. A few weeks later, my annual pediatrician appointment involved the dreaded "getting on a scale." My pediatrician emphatically pronounced that I was 60 pounds overweight and I remember her telling me I would never be able to lose the weight. Those were harsh words to hear as a 15-year-old. I am not sure why she said that to me, but in hindsight, maybe she knew me better than I knew myself. That summer, I set out to prove her wrong.

Initially, my plan involved consuming 1000–1200 calories daily. I often found myself hungry, so I started experimenting with eating more. I added more nutritious foods and increased my caloric intake to approximately 1400–1600 calories per day, but I started ending my meals earlier than usual and waiting as long as I could the next day before eating breakfast. Intermittent fasting was not even a thing back then; in reality, I was just trying to find a way to eat a little more and still lose weight. I soon discovered that my plan was working. That summer, I lost 30 pounds.

It wasn't until I studied Biochemistry in medical school that I discovered why intermittent fasting is such an effective weight loss and maintenance mechanism. Eventually, I managed to lose 70 pounds by the time I graduated and have kept my weight stable since then. We now know that there are many benefits to fasting and I believe it's what has helped me stay relatively healthy in my 50s with no medical problems or any prescription medications.

The Science Behind Fasting

Our body's ultimate goal is always survival, ensuring that all cells are fueled at all times. When we don't eat, it still needs to provide fuel to cells so they can survive. The easiest way to provide fuel to cells is through the food we eat. Our gut breaks down the food and the glucose is transported to our cells with the help of insulin. Without insulin, glucose cannot enter cells. Insulin functions as a lock and key facilitator of glucose transport into cells. When your body runs out of external food sources, insulin levels drop. When insulin levels become very low, it stimulates you by making you hungry, so you can eat and fuel cells again through external glucose sources. Hunger is your body's way of having an easy and steady source of fuel for cells. But … here's the trick: the body has two backup mechanisms besides external glucose from food to ensure that cells are fed. These backup mechanisms require slightly more energy, so your body will always choose easy access to glucose from food first. Remember, our ancestors didn't have access to readily available food and their bodies often tapped into these secondary, backup mechanisms of fuel for cells. I call these backup mechanisms Plan B and Plan C.

Plan B

If you stop eating, your ready supply of external glucose is now gone, but … your cells still need energy and your body still needs to provide it.

Initially, your body waits to see if you'll provide more glucose through food. So, it will wait for a few hours in hopeful anticipation of another easy meal for the cells. Once insulin has dropped to very low levels, usually 4–5 hours after you've eaten, hunger sensations emerge. If you eat, your body once again utilizes the food you've eaten and provides glucose to cells. If you don't eat, your body waits a bit longer, hoping you'll feed it. After approximately 8 hours, your body gets ready for Plan B, which is switching to fuel sources from internal "glucose" storage. Glycogen is a substance stored in the liver that breaks down into glucose when we need it. There are roughly 1000 calories of stored liver glycogen. After approximately 8 hours of not eating, your body now recognizes that it needs to find an alternate method to fuel cells. Instead of releasing insulin, it starts to release a different substance called glucagon.

Glucagon and insulin have opposing functions, and are possibly even "rivals" within the system. Both are secreted by the pancreas, but in opposing directions. Glucagon's function is to stimulate the liver to release its glycogen stores to break them down into glucose. This process is called **glycogenolysis** or, as I like to call it, "Plan B."

You might have noticed this when you get hungry just before you sleep, but if you ignore the hunger and go to bed without eating, you wake up the following morning and find that you're not ravenous, as you would have expected to be. That's because, during the night, your body has switched to Plan B, where it's now using another means of providing cells with glucose.

To better understand this, hypothetically, let's say you stop eating after a 6 p.m. dinner. Your body will switch to glycogen breakdown at around 2 a.m. (Glycogenolysis starts approximately 8 hours after the last meal.) Your body takes roughly 6 hours to burn through all the stored glycogen. That means that around 8 a.m. or so, your body has utilized all of the stored glycogen. If you still don't eat, now your body must find another way to fuel the cells and keep you going. Fortunately, it has a Plan C, which is the next step of the fasting process. It will move on to this a few hours after burning through the glycogen if no other energy source is supplied.

Plan C—Ketosis Gets Those Fat Cells Moving

Plan C involves making "fuel" for cells by tapping into another source and this time, the body turns to fat. The process of making glucose from fat is called gluconeogenesis. This process burns fat cells, which is what many people know as

ketosis. Fat cells are essentially ketone bodies, and it takes a minimum of 16 hours for most people to get into ketosis, so you need to fast for at least this long to start breaking down fat cells. In some individuals, the body doesn't turn to fat burning until 18–19 hours. Fat cells are an amazing fuel source for your cells and a much better fuel for your brain cells than glucose.

So, if you've been fasting for 16–19 hours, your body is now starting to use up fat cells to fuel all the cells in your body, including your brain cells. People in this state of ketosis, where they depend on fat cells for fuel, find that they can think much more clearly and function very well, even though they haven't had any food. It's often a misconception when people say, "I haven't eaten anything and I have brain fog." Brain fog occurs in individuals whose bodies have relied solely on glucose fuels for so long that they are craving this easy fuel. It can sometimes be viewed as a form of "glucose withdrawal" and it can take several weeks for the body to get accustomed to this new way of fueling. This fog usually disappears once the body is accustomed to "intermittent eating" and becomes more efficient at switching to Plans B and C more readily.

Reaching a state of ketosis from fasting can improve your cognitive function, and people who have been fasting for prolonged periods and have made this a normal part of their lifestyle usually find that they are very clear in the mornings while fueling on ketones from ketosis.

Many individuals also report that they are no longer as hungry, since their bodies have now learned to more efficiently switch to these secondary reserve sources of fuel. Be mindful that if you want to lose weight, intermittent fasting is not a free-for-all food fest during the 6–8 hours of eating window, but a way to eat healthy, sustainable meals during a specific period and allow the body to tap into the glycogen and fat stores once it goes into Plan B and Plan C.

So What Are the Actual Benefits of Fasting?

Prevention of Fatty Liver and Insulin Resistance

Plan B benefits: Regularly allowing your body to tap into its glycogen stores prevents an excess glycogen buildup in the liver. When your body is constantly fueling on external glucose, your body is never able to tap into these glycogen stores. Glycogen overload can build up and lead to a condition called fatty liver. Furthermore, eating all day can cause an excess amount of glucose and hence, insulin production. Keep in mind that insulin is also a fat-storage hormone, and while one of its functions is to help transport glucose into cells, it also promotes fat cells to take on excess glucose. Additionally, cells start to not respond as well to insulin if they are "seeing it all day" and begin to become resistant to its effects. This causes more glucose to stay in the bloodstream and also starts the cascade of insulin resistance, prediabetes, and diabetes.

Weight Loss and Clear Cognitive Function

Plan C benefits: Think of the ketone fueling like the gasoline for your car: you can choose to fuel it with regular gasoline— the glucose that comes from food or alternatively, you can fuel it with premium gasoline—the higher-grade fuel of ketosis. A more purified gasoline helps your car run better and the same goes for your body when it comes to ketosis. If you're eating sensibly during your eating windows, ketosis allows your cells to benefit from this cleaner fuel, causing improvement of brain fog, memory, and cognitive function. Fat burning and ketosis also lead to weight loss. More details on this later.

Immune Benefits

Ketosis through fasting also induces two processes that help our immune system: autophagy and apoptosis. These two important processes are what really propel your immune health to the next level.

Apoptosis means killing of cells, and **autophagy** means eating up of one's cells. These processes might seem harmful, but they are actually healthy for your body. Most cells have a lifespan of approximately 90 days, and new cells are constantly being made to replace them. The process of autophagy is how your body gets rid of old cells and cellular debris that are no longer needed. Intermittent fasting stimulates this process and effectively helps your body eliminate dying cells. It also helps to get rid of dysfunctional cells that may have gone awry or have the potential to become cancerous.

Another way I like to explain the process of autophagy is by comparing it to putting your phone in low battery mode. When your phone's battery gets low and you don't have access to a charger, you put it in low battery mode to preserve function for the most vital functions. This is also how autophagy works. When your body realizes that it's not getting enough food, it starts to kill off unwanted, dying, and dysfunctional cells so it doesn't have to waste energy on them. Think of this low battery mode as "spring cleaning" of cells. Your body starts looking at cells thinking, "Hmm, this cell is getting a little old; I'm going to get rid of it" or, "that cell is starting to look dysfunctional; let me get rid of that one too."

This process benefits your immune system because it eliminates dysfunctional and old cells, while focusing energy on the important, healthy new cells.

When you're fasting and in ketosis, not only are you burning fat, using it for fuel and starting to lose weight, but you're stimulating the immune benefits related to autophagy, which usually kick in after 20 hours of fasting. At 24 hours, your body is highly likely to be in autophagy mode. I recommend you fast for 24 hours at least once per month to spring-clean your cells.

While some recommend prolonged fasting, I do not recommend unsupervised fasting of more than 36 hours because the body starts to utilize muscle for fuel, leading to muscle loss. You also don't want to fast for 24 hours consistently as the body may lower metabolism, thinking it's in a fight-or-flight situation and needs to conserve fat cells. Prolonged fasting can also affect fertility or disrupt hormonal levels in females. Many females in my practice are reluctant to try fasting because of a misconception that it can affect their hormonal levels. I have found that when done reasonably without severe caloric restriction and the time restrictions are between 16 and 18 hours, there are no effects on fertility or menopause. The key here is to avoid eliciting stress-inducing chronic cortisol production from severe caloric restriction or prolonged fasting hours.

Some studies have even shown that fasting, when done sensibly in patients with polycystic ovarian syndrome, can improve fertility and, in postmenopausal women, can decrease the incidence of breast cancer.

Intermittent Fasting and Its Impact on Gut Health

In addition to the benefits of Plans B and C, intermittent fasting also has great benefits for your gut. Your gut does much more than just digesting food. It's responsible for helping to make neurotransmitters, producing vitamins, maintaining and repairing the gut lining, and a myriad of other things. If it has to focus on handling food all day, it will be difficult to find time to do anything else and if it can't tend to the other tasks, they'll keep piling up, causing more damage to gut cells.

Studies have also found that having nutrients available only periodically can trigger adaptive responses that make the gut barrier stronger and more functional. This reduces your risk of developing a leaky gut and ensures that harmful substances get passed out of the body instead of into your bloodstream. A sort of survival of the fittest phenomenon.

Types of Fasts and How to Start

There are a few different types of fasts. One is the 16:8 method, where you fast for 16 hours, and then eat during an 8-hour window. You can extend this to 18:6 or even 20:4, although I don't recommend the latter to women.

When undertaking a time-restricted fast, I recommend eating two meals, and a snack, or even just two meals. Many people do not need a full three meals every day unless they are underweight. Make your meals at least 70% plant-based for maximum effectiveness, with only around 30% "other," which can come in the form of clean sources of animal protein or other complex carbohydrates. While I don't like to restrict any specific foods, avoiding refined carbohydrates should be the goal. That being said, I know that diet should also not be a static, rigid intake of only these foods and I believe that if you follow this healthy eating plan 80% of the time, your body is capable of dealing with the occasional dietary detour. Also, ensure you're getting enough protein from either your plant-based options or animal sources.

Remember, intermittent fasting is not a pass to eat anything you like during the unrestricted period. It is still important to make healthy decisions and eat a balanced choice of two healthy meals that are predominantly plant-based (and incorporate proteins in the form of plant proteins or clean animal proteins), while enjoying some healthy carbohydrates in smaller portions. You can even have the occasional treat after a meal. While we know the benefits of ketosis are great for the body and the brain, we want to induce ketosis through fasting, rather than strictly high-fat/protein keto foods, which do not provide your gut with the food those beneficial gut microbes love to feast on.

There are other types of intermittent fasting including 5:2-day fasts, which involve eating sensibly throughout the day for 5 days followed by 2 days of restricting eating to once a day and approximately 500 calories. Alternate-day fasts work in a similar manner, but you're alternating days of regular eating with eating once a day for only 500 calories. While some studies show that these effectively improve insulin sensitivity and weight loss, I do not recommend they become part of a routine regimen for women since they may induce a cortisol stress response that can affect hormones or fertility. Occasionally, they may be fine.

TIMELINE OF
FASTING

16-20 HOURS

Glycogen stores are depleted and the body starts to turn to fat cells for fuel. (Start of ketosis)

4-6 HOURS

After last meal, insulin levels drop and hunger is stimulated.

24-36 HOURS

Autophagy is maximized, but risk of muscle loss can start after 36 hours.

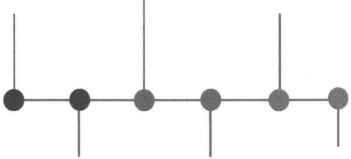

36 HOURS

(Prolonged fasts) Should only be done with prolonged fasting eating protocols (fasting mimicking diets) and under medical supervision to avoid muscle loss.

8-10 HOURS

Glucagon is released by the pancreas and stimulates the start of glycogen burning in the liver.

20-24 HOURS

Ketosis continues and the process of autophagy starts.

If your goal is weight loss, I don't usually recommend counting calories, but first, see how you do during the first week of fasting. Most people who follow this ratio will lose weight without counting calories, but if you have not lost weight, counting calories for a couple of weeks should help you understand what your body needs. Most people can lose weight by consuming 1300–1600 calories of the above ratio of foods if they fast for a 16–18-hour period.

Try to avoid eating 4 hours before sleep so that Plans B and C can kick in more effectively during the night.

Remember, fasting requires some mental discipline and a structured approach to life, which can also help with other areas. It increases your mindfulness and improves your overall quality of life, encouraging you to think more about your wellness and prioritize looking after yourself.

Things to Remember

- **Fasting** can boost gut health through enhanced microbial diversity, improved gut barrier function, and reduced inflammation.

- **Intermittent fasting and time-restricted feeding** are your body's way of tapping into healthier mechanisms. When you feel hungry, it's not your body saying, "You need to eat right now," it's your body saying, "If I don't get an easy fuel source, I'm going to move on to Plans B and C as fuel sources."

- **During your eating window,** eat only two meals or two meals and one snack, with a 70% plant-based focus. Good snack ideas include a Greek-style yogurt with some fruit, a handful of nuts, or a fruit smoothie.

- **If you're considering fasting,** no matter what type of intermittent fasting you settle on, it's good to start by discussing your plan with a doctor, and getting bloodwork done to make sure there aren't any contraindications. Having the bloodwork done at the start will also make it easier to monitor your progress.

- **Start small with fasting,** and begin with short fasts. Try eating during a 12-hour window for a week, and then progress to 10 hours a day and then 8 hours daily. If the goal is weight loss, remember that some people don't tap into fat-burning mode before 18–20 hours, so you might have to experiment to see which time restriction you respond to. Gradually increase your fasting duration over time. Don't try to do an extensive fast when you're used to eating three meals a day, plus snacks. You'll shock your body and may make yourself ill.
- **Keep a journal** to track how fasting impacts your gut health and overall well-being.

FAQs

1. Can I have coffee in the morning and still remain in ketosis mode?

Yes, as long as it's black coffee. If you must have milk in your coffee, a dash (less than 1 TBS of heavy cream) can keep you in ketosis. Why heavy cream? It has zero carbs and less than 50 calories, so it will not take you out of ketosis. Also, many people will find that it is filling because of its high-fat content. If you are lactose intolerant, you can try coconut milk or other nondairy milk, but keep it under 50 calories so you don't take your body out of a ketotic state.

2. Why don't I just eat a high keto diet?

Studies have shown that while high-fat/animal protein keto diets help with weight loss, many restrict plant-based foods essential for the growth and maintenance of beneficial gut bacteria. Carnivore-type diets are presumed to be mostly animal protein-based, but studies show that our ancestors actually ate a lot more plant-based foods than presumed, including fruits and vegetables that were in season. The fiber in these foods is feeding them, NOT you. So, while the benefits of ketosis from a keto-type diet are okay as a temporary 30–60-day kickstart to weight loss, it's better to induce ketosis (fat burning) from intermittent fasting (Plan C) than to opt for a strictly keto diet.

3. Is fasting beneficial for everyone or should some people avoid it?

While fasting is good for most people, always check with your doctor before starting an intermittent fasting regimen. Intermittent fasting should not be done if you are underweight, have an eating disorder, or are an insulin-dependent diabetic. Most individuals who are prediabetic or have mild diabetes can safely start a fasting regimen, but should do so under the supervision of a doctor.

4. Can I exercise if I am fasting?

Yes, but be mindful of ensuring adequate food quantities, especially if you're a professional athlete. If you're not a professional athlete and want to ramp up fat burning, exercise right before you break your fast. The extra energy needed to supply muscles utilizes more fat cells and may allow a more accelerated switch to autophagy.

CHAPTER 6

Weight Loss and the Gut

The Skinny on the Gut–Weight Axis

L osing weight can help transform your gut; transforming your gut can help you lose weight. Both alter your gut microbiome for the better. In this chapter, we're going to look at the fascinating connections between the gut and appetite regulation and insulin sensitivity.

The Role of Gut Microbes in Metabolism and Appetite Regulation

We've already explored the analogy of beneficial bacteria as helpful, productive employees, and harmful bacteria as unhelpful ones. The beneficial bacteria create some really useful byproducts while they're "on the clock"—from **psychobiotics** (neurotransmitters) to other postbiotics like short-chain fatty acids (SCFAs). One type of postbiotic, called butyrate, is key to helping control your appetite. Butyrate is responsible for satiety-signaling. It affects certain receptors called GLP-1 receptors, telling your body it's full. If that sounds familiar, it's because GLP-1 is the same receptor that certain injectable weight loss medications also work on. These medications are intended for individuals with diabetes, but they were discovered to help decrease appetite and cause weight loss due to their effect on these receptors. Another way that our gut microbes work on weight loss is by releasing a peptide called PYY. PYY sends direct signals to our brain's appetite center, turning it off when our gut microbes are full. In other words, when they're full, you're full too!

The more plant-based fibers and probiotic foods you eat, the more butyrate you produce, and the more GLP-1 and PYY you'll activate.

One of the gut bacteria that is particularly recognized for stimulating GLP-1 is called Akkermansia. People who are overweight often have deficiencies of Akkermansia in their gut. Non-overweight individuals generally have much higher levels of both Bifidobacteria and Akkermansia. It's no coincidence. Both of these bacteria affect the appetite center of the individual and ensure that the appetite gets "turned off" when the person has had enough to eat.

Think of them like a team. Bifidobacterium, Lactobacillus, and Akkermansia are players that get along and work well together. The more they network and collaborate with one another, the better off your body will be. Similarly, if you recruit certain "bad" gut bacteria to the team, they will stimulate your appetite, and make it much more difficult for you to avoid overeating. They literally "hijack" your eating behaviors.

Remember, different microbes produce different postbiotics, so diversity is key here.

So, how do you get these bacteria, and how can you increase the levels if you are deficient? Eating a variety of foods that they love such as moderate amounts of inulin-rich vegetables. These include food such as asparagus, chicory root, and artichokes. Tuber and root vegetables such as sweet potatoes, taro, turnips, and beetroot are also great sources of fiber for your gut players. Akkermansia in particular also love eating foods such as pomegranates, cranberries, and unpeeled apples. Akkermansia particularly enjoy apple skins, so you can encourage their growth by eating organic, unpeeled apples. The common adage of "an apple a day keeps the doctor away" may have been more accurate than previously presumed. Is it possible that our ancestors knew a lot more about natural therapies than we do now?

Balance Is Key

Firmicutes are bacteria that need to be cautiously balanced in the gut. A high ratio of Firmicutes in relation to Bifidobacteria can cause an imbalance in the gut. People who are heavy meat eaters and who don't consume enough plant-based foods put themselves at risk of high Firmicutes to Bifidobacterium ratios, and this may increase the risk of colon cancer. However, having a reverse ratio of these microbes has been shown to be beneficial. Adding animal protein in smaller amounts creates a good Firmicutes/Bifidobacterium ratio. Combining foods like yogurt with berries and apples, for example, can help get the party going in the gut.

Your gut bacteria are also important when it comes to regulating fat storage and keeping your metabolism balanced. These bacteria help synthesize essential vitamins like vitamin K and certain B vitamins, which are integral in keeping your metabolism in check.

There is sometimes a tug-of-war between your gut microbes and your body as to who will receive calories first. In a study published in the journal "Natural Communications," two groups of dieters were compared, and consumption of the same number of calories was present in both groups. The participants who followed a high-fiber diet "lost" 216 calories compared to those on a processed food diet, who "lost" 116 calories despite being on similar calorie restrictions. More importantly, the fiber-rich group lost slightly more weight than the other group and had higher reports of "not feeling hungry."

Let's explore this further. Processed foods tend to be absorbed higher in your gastrointestinal tract, leaving less nutrition for the gut microbes lower down in your gut. These beneficial microbes that help with appetite regulation produce important postbiotics that affect your sense of satiety. They need fiber to do it. They won't produce the postbiotics that make you feel full if they don't get enough plant-based fiber. When they are satisfied, so are you.

Some studies have shown us that the gut microbiota composition differs between obese and lean individuals. Similar to the abnormal cancer ratio, individuals with BMIs in the obesity range often have a higher proportion of Firmicutes and a lower proportion of Bacteroidetes than lean individuals. This further indicates that there's a close connection between your gut bacteria and your body weight. This cause–effect relationship also points to a potential role of gut microbiota in weight management.

It's also interesting to note that your gut microbiota may affect how you perceive tastes. Studies suggest that certain harmful microbes can alter the activity of taste receptors, which may influence our food preferences and contribute to unhealthy eating behaviors.

Gut Health and Insulin Sensitivity

Tied in with this are the insulin levels we discussed in the chapter on fasting. If you aren't fasting and you eat all day (say from around 7 a.m. to 9 p.m.), insulin will be released throughout the day, which means that your pancreas, which is responsible for insulin production, has to constantly work to pump out insulin with every meal.

Think of this as a situation similar to "The Boy Who Cried Wolf." If you're unfamiliar with the fable, this refers to a shepherd boy who repeatedly fooled the villagers into thinking a wolf was attacking his flock. When an actual wolf finally did appear, the villagers ignored the boy's calls for help because he had tricked them too many times and the wolf ended up eating the sheep (and in some versions, also the boy).

This is a useful way to look at insulin resistance and insulin sensitivity. Insulin resistance means your cells are unresponsive to insulin's actions. If the cells that are utilizing glucose for fuel see insulin too many times a day, they become less responsive to insulin and start resisting its effects, hence the term "insulin resistance." This can start the cascade of pre-diabetes and diabetes. When cells become resistant to insulin, less glucose is properly transported into the cells for fuel, leading to more glucose in the bloodstream.

Stress also plays a role in insulin sensitivity because your body responds to stress similarly: it will handle it well when exposed to it occasionally, but will handle it poorly if you become chronically stressed. When you're chronically stressed, your body releases more insulin and cortisol as a protective mechanism to help you store fat (to prepare you to survive whatever it perceives as stressful). This process also contributes to insulin resistance.

Of course, what you eat is also very significant here. Certain bacteria, such as Akkermansia and Bifidobacterium, are associated with improved insulin sensitivity and higher metabolic profiles—mostly because of the type of postbiotics they release.

Harmful microbes are another factor. They can contribute to inflammation and insulin resistance, making you more likely to develop diabetes. The more "good guys" you can invite to your team by eating healthy, whole, unprocessed foods, the less space there is for these harmful microbes, and the better you're likely to feel. Having a balanced and diverse gut microbiota is key to metabolic health and insulin sensitivity.

Remember, all beneficial microbes have different jobs and must be present to do those jobs. The team of employees has a range of skills and everyone performs a unique task. If you don't have the right team of employees, the individual tasks don't get done, the team can't work well together, and systems stop working efficiently.

Exercise, Gut Health, and Weight Loss

It's already well established that physical activity can improve your weight management and help you slim down, but not many people are aware that exercise also has a pretty big impact on your gut health. Exercise has been shown to alter the composition and diversity of your gut microbiome, which will increase the number of beneficial bacteria.

Doing regular aerobic exercise is particularly associated with increased gut microbial diversity and could offer some major benefits when it comes to weight management. Exercise may also increase the production of SCFAs, improving your metabolic health and weight control.

Exercise doesn't have to be intense to be beneficial. Doing just 20–30 minutes each day for 5 days a week—even if you're just walking—is beneficial. That's particularly true if you walk immediately after eating because that quickly utilizes the glucose you've consumed to help your body supply oxygen and nutrients to your muscles. Walking after meals has also been shown to stabilize your blood glucose levels.

The Sleep–Weight Connection: How Sleep Affects Your Immune System and Your Weight

Remember that your gut is performing some significant roles while you're asleep, so not sleeping enough can affect its ability to perform these tasks.

Sleep alters the production of two hormones: **leptin** and **ghrelin**. Leptin is a hormone that your fat cells produce. It works a bit like an appetite suppressant. Your brain's satiety signaling is affected by leptin levels. Ghrelin is a hormone that increases your appetite. Sleep deprivation is thought to increase your levels of ghrelin and lower your levels of leptin, making it more difficult for you to control your appetite. It also prompts you to reach for high-energy, sugary foods. With lower levels of leptin, you're less likely to feel full and satisfied, and may continue eating when you don't need to. Higher levels of ghrelin also hijack your satiety signaling. I like to use the term, "The sleep gremlins are making more ghrelin."

Historically speaking, we are less likely to resist poor food choices when we're sleep-deprived because again, the survival mechanism in our body kicks in and if your body thinks you're in a stressful situation, it will generate that fight or flight response, which will cause you to eat more (to save energy for the perceived threat causing you to not sleep). Willpower has no chance with ghrelin and leptin.

Developing a Personalized Gut Health Plan for Weight Loss

Everyone's microbiome is unique, almost like a fingerprint. No two individuals will have identical microbiomes and you need to eat different foods to support your unique blueprint.

We also need to recognize that different people have different needs. Demographically speaking, the gut microbiome of someone living in Africa is very different from that of someone living in North America, and we still don't understand all the intricacies involved in these differences. This is why a one-size-fits-all approach is never the answer and why I ultimately look deeply at a gut analysis to determine what's going on internally.

Interestingly, the body will also make us hungry when it is in need of certain nutrients that are essential for making important neurotransmitters. Dr. Braverman is a psychiatrist who developed a gut–brain assessment that recognizes that we all make four major neurotransmitters that affect our personality: **acetylcholine, dopamine, GABA,** and **serotonin**. While we all produce these four neurotransmitters, we each make them in varying quantities, and they actually have a big impact on our personalities and how we interact with the world. For example, my husband is an ICU doctor, and one of the most important aspects of his job is being able to remain calm in a high-stress environment. He is able to do so because he is GABA-natured, meaning he produces more of the neurotransmitter GABA, which promotes calmness and relaxation. GABA-natured individuals tend to be reliable and work well under pressure. Other individuals have different personality traits based on which neurotransmitter they make more of. If you are acetylcholine-natured—as am I, you like to multitask and get things done quickly but can be a little impatient at times. Acetylcholine-dominant people tend to be efficient and like to complete tasks quickly, without wasting time. They may not be as calm as GABA-dominant folks, but they are often proactive and productive individuals who are always looking to move forward. Many people (often women) who multitask well are acetylcholine-dominant. Acetylcholine is the neurotransmitter that helps nerve impulses travel quickly. It doesn't mean that they're more intelligent—but they have faster reflexes and might be able to get more accomplished in a shorter time than others. Acetylcholine-dominant individuals can often be "out-of-the-box" thinkers.

Another example would be a serotonin-dominant individual. Remember that serotonin is the neurotransmitter that helps elevate your mood and keep you happy. These people tend to be "life lovers," who constantly want to explore, travel, and revel in their freedom. They often dislike being tied down and are full of energy and cheerfulness. They are often amazing people with whom to socialize and tend to have a contagious, happy spirit.

Finally, there's the dopamine-dominant individual. Dopamine is our excitatory neurotransmitter, which means that it triggers a sense of excitement. Dopamine-dominant people tend to be energetic and competitive and are frequently driven to rise to the top. If you know go-getters who have a lot of inner drive, they may be dopamine-dominant individuals.

It's important to start with understanding where your dominance lies and what that means about who you are. Deficiency in any of these neurotransmitters can occur, especially if you're not eating foods containing the building blocks of these neurotransmitters. Not making enough of a specific neurotransmitter can cause symptoms such as depression, anxiety, and brain fog. Deficiencies of these neurotransmitters can make us hungry as the body tries to replenish low levels by "demanding" certain foods, in order to make more of these neurotransmitters. Many times, especially when deficiencies are very low, the body craves "quick-fix" junk foods in an attempt to quickly increase the low levels. We will discuss this further in Chapter 9.

It's likely that in the next few years, we'll see much more information about these unique gut–brain nutrient deficiencies that will revolutionize personalized treatments. This book aims to give you a head-start on that information.

Things to Remember

- **Gut bacteria play a significant role in metabolism and appetite regulation,** which can influence body weight.
- **Gut health affects insulin sensitivity,** meaning it has implications in obesity and diabetes.
- **Gut microbiome diversity** is crucial for weight management.
- **Balance is key** when it comes to certain bacteria like Akkermansia and Firmicutes. Too much of these two bacteria may not be a good thing, so a delicate balance is key. There is so much we are still learning about the gut and why the diversity of plant-based foods and the microbiome is important.
- **Exercise can improve gut health** and support weight control.
- **Lack of sleep** can thwart your weight loss goals.
  Short-term inflammation and cortisol release are necessary and helpful. Chronic release is not.

Work on managing chronic stress and sleep deprivation to avoid chronic inflammation and resistance to weight loss.

- **A personalized approach is critical** for leveraging gut health for weight loss.

  Be patient and consistent in your efforts to improve gut health. While gut health can significantly improve in 30 days, it may take longer in some individuals. Other conditions such as food allergies, inflammatory bowel disease, and IBS could be present, so it's important to report any symptoms to your doctor.

- **Consider doing a microbiome analysis** to look for gut dysbiosis and any unhealthy inflammatory findings.

CHAPTER 7

That Gut Feeling

The Gut–Brain Connection

That "gut feeling" is something we have all experienced and the science behind it proves that it's not just in our imagination.

The Vagus Nerve and Gut–Brain Communication

The vagus nerve is the super highway of gut–brain communication. It is the longest cranial nerve and links the gut to the brain and the brain to the gut. It serves as an incredibly powerful two-way messaging platform that can pass messages back and forth, allowing these two body parts to communicate. The vagus nerve forms the foundation of the gut–brain axis.

A fascinating study undertaken on mice has confirmed this. Mice are often used in studies as stand-ins for humans because the mouse metabolism and physiology resemble that of humans, and their relatively short lifespan means it's easy to see cause and effect more rapidly.

During the study, scientists severed the nerve connection between the gut and the brain, but they left the connection between the brain and the gut intact. That meant that the brain could send messages to the gut, but the gut couldn't send messages to the brain. The experiment had some pretty astonishing results; the mice stopped showing signs of fear. The results were repeatable, which confirms that the gut certainly sends messages to the brain that affect the brain's behavior. It also confirms that at least some of those messages have a big impact on how we feel and behave. You've probably heard of the term "gut sense or a gut feeling." Well, it's a real phenomenon.

Your "gut sense" is a sensation triggered by your gut in response to perceived threats. Your gut takes note of your surroundings and sends nerve signals to your brain that you might not even be consciously aware of. A smell could be enough to set it off, but so could a million other tiny factors that you might not have noticed consciously—and that's often why the "gut sense" is often dismissed. We don't have a rational explanation for why we feel that something is off; we just do—the same way that a mouse might feel uneasy when in the vicinity of a cat, even if its conscious brain hasn't yet detected the cat's presence.

As we can see from the study with the mice, animals clearly possess this ability, and it's thought to be much stronger in them than in humans—perhaps not surprisingly, since humans often suppress their gut instincts and opt for more logic-based decision-making. However, it's interesting to note that children have a stronger gut sense than adults and that women have stronger gut senses than men.

Learning to Trust Your Gut

Why might a child's gut sense be stronger if an adult has had longer to recognize dangerous cues? It's probably that children operate much more on instinct, the way an animal might, rather than from learned and rationalized responses.

An adult making a decision may create a list of pros and cons based on the things that they have been conditioned to believe from prior experiences, but a child hasn't developed this skill yet, and is much more likely to heed their gut instinct. Women similarly seem to be more in tune with their gut sense and often react more instinctively than men.

Your gut sense can sometimes be too sensitive. If you've dealt with a past trauma in your past such as abuse or a tragic event, your vagus nerve can send too many "something's wrong" signals to the brain. It can trigger a sense of anxiety, making an individual feel uneasy. This is a sort of hyper-response that is stimulated by the body's attempts to protect the individual from harm, but this instinctive feeling is often overwhelming and can make it hard for some individuals to cope.

Many of the decisions we make in life are based on two factors: what you learn from past experiences and your gut instincts. What you learn is really valuable and important up to a point, but it also needs to be coupled with your subconscious warnings and signals so that you can make valid, balanced decisions. Mark Twain famously said, "We should be careful to get out of an experience only the wisdom that is in it and stop there lest we be like the cat that sits down on a hot stove lid. She will never sit down on a hot stove lid again and that is well, but also she will never sit down on a cold one anymore."

Similarly, your subconscious warnings must be tempered with your understanding of the situation and past experiences.

How Managing Your Stress Affects Your Gut

Your body's primary goal is always survival, and your immune system is always looking for the best ways to do that. When your body encounters a situation that triggers stress or a sense of danger, it releases a neurotransmitter called noradrenaline, the fight or flight neurotransmitter.

If you're in the woods and encounter a bear, your body will immediately start releasing noradrenaline. Noradrenaline accelerates the heart rate to increase blood flow to your muscles, allowing them to work harder to help you escape the threat. Noradrenaline simultaneously decreases blood flow to the gut because digesting food isn't high on the list of things you need to do while running away from a bear. Your body wants to devote all of its energy to the act of escaping.

Now here's the thing though, noradrenaline can't be released over prolonged periods; it's designed to be used in short bursts to help us escape from that bear, for example. It also reduces your appetite and stimulates your gut to get rid of anything that is already in it, causing diarrhea. Think of those times you were scared or anxious and had to run to the bathroom. That was noradrenaline in action. Prolonged release of noradrenaline can be a real problem and can be damaging to the heart. Essentially, your body is sensing the stress, causing your heart to continue to work harder and your system to stay in fight or flight mode. It can't do that over prolonged periods, so your body switches over to release of the long-haul stress manager—cortisol.

Cortisol is a stress-related chemical that your body uses for long-term survival. Persistent and chronic cortisol production will promote fat storage as the body thinks it is storing fat for an emergency. Remember, your brain and your body are very intricately linked, so when one becomes stressed, so does the other.

Irritable Bowel Syndrome (IBS): A Gut Problem or a Gut–Brain Problem?

The most prevalent gut disorder is actually a gut–brain disorder and provides more proof of the strong connection between the gut and the brain. IBS is an intestinal motility disorder that can cause either diarrhea (IBS-D), constipation (IBS-C), or a mix of both (IBS-M). Stress and early childhood trauma increase susceptibility to developing it and most sufferers report worsening of their symptoms during periods of stress. When the body is under stress, the vagus nerve sends signals to the brain, which the brain interprets as a reason to get ready for battle. So, instead of a "rest and digest" situation that prevails when we aren't stressed, the body reacts with a "fight or flight" response. This fight or flight leads to a miscommunication between the gut and the brain. In some individuals, it triggers diarrhea, while in some, it triggers constipation or a combination of both. Studies have also illustrated that gut dysbiosis can trigger this miscommunication, most likely due to an effect on the neurotransmitters serotonin and GABA.

What Can You Do About Stress?

Some stress management techniques to improve your gut health and reduce inflammation:

- **Mindfulness-based stress reduction (MBSR):** This technique involves paying attention to your present moment in a nonjudgmental way. You do not judge, analyze, or make any attempt to change your situation; you simply accept it as it is.
- **Practicing gratitude:** Start writing in a daily journal and spend a few minutes reflecting on good things that happened throughout the day or things that you are grateful for. They could be specific or as general as "I am grateful for a roof over my head."
- **Meditation and prayer:** People who pray or meditate have been shown to add an extra 5 years to their lives. Carve out time to make this a regular habit.
- **Focus on the now, not the future:** Anxiety and stress usually occur when you start to worry about what will happen. So instead, focus on the now and not the what-if.
- **Take a relaxing bath:** Warm baths help to relax muscles and ease tension.
- **Call a loved one or friend:** Studies show that spending just 10 minutes connecting with someone can reduce anxiety levels and loneliness.
- **Take a walk or sit outdoors:** Find a temporary activity that distracts you from the stressor until you're more calm and able to handle it. Walking or sitting outdoors can help with this.

Things to Remember

- **The vagus nerve** is the primary communication pathway between the gut and the brain, passing messages in both directions.
- **Manage stress carefully** so that it does not impact your ability to digest food or put your body into long-term survival mode.
- **Choose fermented and fiber-rich foods** to support good gut health and encourage diverse bacteria.

CHAPTER 8

The Gut's Role

In Brain Development and Brain Disorders

If you want to optimize your baby's gut health, start with mom's gut health.

The Gut Microbiome's Impact on Early Brain Development

Studies suggest that a well-populated infant gut is closely related to how well its brain is likely to develop.

Prenatal and early postnatal periods are particularly critical windows for brain development, and a lot of the groundwork for neural connections is being established during these periods. This is also when the gut microbiota starts to flourish, including baby's exposure to microbes during birth and through breastfeeding.

Further research is needed to fully understand this, but several animal studies suggest that the gut can impact neurodevelopment by affecting the production of proteins that support the development of important neural connections.

Gut Bacteria and Cognitive Development in Children: How to Raise a Baby Genius

Cognitive development in children refers to the way in which a child thinks and begins to understand the world. It encompasses skills like problem-solving, decision-making, language learning, memory, and more.

A 2018 study found that children with a higher diversity of gut bacteria scored better on cognitive tests at 2 and 3 years of age. This is likely due to the microbiome's effect on neural signaling pathways.

Neurodevelopment is heavily influenced by short-chain fatty acids (SCFAs), which, as we previously discussed, are the postbiotics made by our beneficial bacteria. Fat plays an important part in a baby's brain development, and that's one of the reasons breast milk is so good for babies. Breast milk is rich in beneficial fats and omega-3 fatty acids. Formula also contains a good amount of fat and is designed to mimic breast milk and help a baby's brain develop, so if you're a mom who cannot breastfeed for reasons beyond your control, don't worry. However, I encourage all moms who are able to breastfeed to do so, even if it's just for a few weeks.

The beneficial fats present in breast milk are called human milk oligosaccharides (HMOs). HMOs stimulate the production of some healthy bacteria in the gut, and increase the number of SCFAs. HMOs also feed a specific strain of Bifidobacterium called Bifidobacterium breve, which has been shown to have immense immune-boosting benefits for babies. Another interesting study showed that infants who excelled at point and gaze, the ability to closely follow an object, and a predictor of higher intelligence also had higher levels of Bifidobacterium in their gut. SCFAs stimulate the production of certain neurotransmitters, including GABA, which helps with brain development. SCFAs also have positive impacts on the hippocampus, the learning and memory center. Not surprisingly, breastfed babies have up to 7 points higher on the IQ scale and appear to have better educational achievements later in life.

Colonization of an infant's gut occurs even before the neurological system is fully developed, so moms, what you eat while you're pregnant does matter.

Sometimes, a baby's microbiome can be a little "off" due to multiple factors, such as premature birth, frequent antibiotic use in the mom, nonvaginal births, lack of breastfeeding, etc. Some studies have shown that when babies are born through the vaginal canal, they come into contact with beneficial bacteria, which they can use to start building up their own microbiome. Obviously, some of these factors are not in your control, but it's important to recognize all the factors affecting a baby's gut microbiome, so we can give a baby's immune system the best start possible.

Factors that can affect a baby's gut microbiome:

- *Premature births*
- *Frequent antibiotic use*
- *C-section births*
- *Lack of breastfeeding*

If for any reason, a baby's birth does not have these optimal circumstances, here are a few ways to strengthen baby's gut microbiome:

- Breastfeed
- Consider delaying your baby's first bath for 24 hours after birth
- Encourage skin-to-skin contact with baby

The Gut Microbiome's Influence on Learning and Memory

We are mostly dependent on animal studies to understand how the gut affects learning and memory. Germ-free mice have been used to show us that the gut influences memory. In studies specifically done to assess memory, the germ-free mice had significantly impaired memory when compared with conventional mice. Interestingly, introducing healthy microbes to these germ-free mice saw these effects partially reverse.

Can having insufficient beneficial gut bacteria during these early stages affect a baby's brain? Pregnant women and infants who were given a long course of antibiotics showed a measurable decrease in certain beneficial bacteria. When penicillin derivatives were used, they decreased two important bacteria: Bifidobacterium and Lactobacillus. This is not to deter anyone from taking antibiotics if they are necessary—it's just a reminder that if we deplete these microbes, we need to replenish them, or compensate for the loss. That might mean bumping up your intake of fermented foods or taking probiotics after a course of antibiotics.

Gut Bacteria's Impact on Mood Disorders and Anxiety

Various studies have shown links between gut microbiota and certain mental health conditions, including depression and anxiety.

GABA, a neurotransmitter that helps us feel calm, can make us start to feel anxious if levels become deficient. If the gut employees aren't being fed the right foods, they aren't going to be able to make the products you need. If, for example, you're not eating the precursor foods that help you produce GABA (foods rich in glutamic acid) or the precursor food that help you make serotonin (tryptophan-rich foods), you're not going to be producing the neurotransmitters that you need to keep your mood up and your anxiety down. Serotonin, which is key to this and is predominantly made in the gut—has an enormous impact on your mood. We will discuss this further in Chapter 9.

A 2011 study found that *Lactobacillus rhamnosus*, a beneficial gut bacteria, reduced anxiety-like behavior in mice because it appeared to modulate their GABA and serotonin levels.

The Gut Microbiome and Neurodegenerative Diseases

There's also some evidence to suggest that the microbes in your gut protect you from neurodegenerative diseases. Alzheimer's, for example, sees the formation of amyloid plaques, which are inflammatory plaques that prevent neuronal connections. The first areas that tend to be affected are the parts of the brain that work on memory. We don't fully understand why these areas are most affected, but a lot of research has been done to understand where these plaques come from and what they are doing in the brain. So far, we have established that they are inflammatory in nature and travel to the brain from the gut. Now, scientists are finding that the diversity of the gut organisms in Alzheimer's patients is lower than in individuals who don't have Alzheimer's. It's thought that this lack of diversity signifies gut inflammation, sending signals through the vagus nerve into the brain. These signals are protein signals that transport plaque-like deposits.

The sequence of events is believed to be as follows:

- Decreased number of beneficial gut microbes leads to a decreased gut diversity.
- This causes weakening of the gut lining and an overabundance of bad gut microbes, which release inflammatory toxins, leading to inflammation.
- The inflammation is released systemically through communication pathways to the brain.
- The inflammation is deposited in the brain in the form of plaques that cause a breakdown in neuronal communications.

To remove or prevent further inflammation in the brain, you have to decrease the inflammation in the gut. One way to do this is to increase gut diversity by increasing your intake of plant-based foods to 25–30 per week.

Alcohol is another substance that is thought to increase the risk of Alzheimer's because it can kill off beneficial microbes. Think about the alcohol present in hand sanitizer that is used to kill viruses and bacteria on your hands, and then compare that with consumed alcohol entering your gut. It will inevitably destroy some of the beneficial microorganisms. Artificial sugars are similarly harmful, including artificial sweeteners and high fructose corn syrup, which is found in a lot of processed foods. High fructose corn syrup feeds harmful bacteria, and artificial sweeteners weaken the gut lining. Table sugar can also do this. Many believe that sugar is a natural substance and not harmful, but the sugar of today is highly processed and not the same as the sugar of our ancestors, which was derived from unrefined sugarcane.

Research has also discovered that altering your gut microbiota could contribute to the development of other neurodegenerative diseases, such as Parkinson's. It's thought that the gut can influence neurodegeneration through metabolic interactions and direct neurosignaling.

Autism is also an interesting area to explore in terms of gut diversity. Some links have been made between the most debilitating symptoms of autism (social withdrawal, inability to recognize and give social cues, lethargy, etc.) and poor gut diversity. There appears to be a correlation between the gut's diversity and an individual's ability to cope in these areas. Interestingly, it's been noted that when autistic patients eat diets rich in fiber and fermented foods, there is visible improvement. Fecal transplants have also shown some success in improving autism symptoms.

Things to Remember

- **The gut can influence** cognitive development, learning, memory, and mood disorders.
- **Alterations in the gut microbiota** may contribute to neurodegenerative diseases. **Optimizing gut health** could benefit cognitive and mental health.
- **Avoiding dysbiosis** can prevent Alzheimer's and other types of dementia and improve neuropsychological conditions.
- **Gut diversity** promotes improvement in gut health. Aim to consume 25–30 different plant-based foods along with a variety of pickled and fermented foods weekly.
- **To boost your Lactobacillus and Bifidobacterium levels,** remember to eat berries, artichokes, asparagus, chicory root, broccoli, lentils, kefir, and Greek-style full-fat yogurt.
- Optimize baby's microbiome by breastfeeding, delaying their first bath, and encouraging skin-to-skin contact.

CHAPTER 9

The Psychobiotic Connection
How Food Affects Your Mood

In previous chapters, we discussed how the gut and the brain communicate with each other through the vagus nerve. Our gut also affects our mood and our personality traits based on the predominance of neurotransmitters we make.

The gut microbiome is teeming with bacteria, fungi, and viruses, all of which coexist and perform different functions. Some of these are responsible for the production of neurochemicals, which the brain uses to regulate mood and cognition. Our body makes more than 50 neurochemicals that affect our nervous system. According to psychiatrist Dr. Eric Braverman, four neurotransmitters can significantly impact our personalities. They can also dictate how we behave and function in different situations based on which ones our body makes more of. These four neurotransmitters are GABA, acetylcholine, dopamine, and serotonin. These are sometimes called psychobiotics and are types of postbiotics.

For example, a strain of Lactobacillus is believed to be involved in the production of GABA, a neurotransmitter that helps to keep us calm. Without enough GABA, an individual can become anxious. GABA also influences sleep and helps with deep sleep quality by regulating Delta sleep waves. If you're not eating foods that support Lactobacillus, you may not be able to make enough GABA.

When beneficial microbes work together, they may also be responsible for making serotonin and other neurotransmitters. We've already explored the importance of several beneficial microbes working together in managing inflammation, but did you know that they are also responsible for making certain neurotransmitters such as serotonin? Serotonin is often called the "happiness chemical" because it's important for mental well-being and mood. Your body needs adequate amounts of Bifidobacterium and Lactobacillus to support its production.

While there's still much to learn about psychobiotics, we know that supporting the right bacteria within the gut can help us combat mental health conditions. Studies have found that individuals who have a diverse composition of beneficial gut microbes are often less anxious and have better mental resilience and well-being.

GABA: The Calming Neurotransmitter

GABA is the neurotransmitter responsible for helping you stay relaxed and calm and it's produced in the brain. If your brain produces more GABA, you are more likely to be a low-stress, calm-under-pressure type of person.

GABA production occurs predominantly in the brain. Approximately 50% of the population are GABA-natured individuals. Their main characteristics are reliability, dedication, and the ability to handle pressure well. GABA-natured individuals are sensible and not prone to fluctuating moods. They tend to be in careers that require people to function well under stress, such as ICU staff, police officers, or emergency medical personnel.

While some people make more GABA than others, anyone can become deficient in this neurotransmitter. If your brain doesn't produce sufficient GABA, you may start to feel anxious and more stressed. GABA is rich in the amino acid glutamic acid, which is found in foods such as fish, nuts, eggs, certain cheeses, and spinach.

Interestingly, another side effect of too little GABA is waking up in the middle of the night because your body won't be able to regulate Delta waves during deep, REM sleep.

If you are a GABA-natured individual and you aren't eating enough foods rich in glutamic acid to support GABA production, you may find that you start to feel a bit "off" and not yourself. You may find that you struggle to relax, even if you are usually a relaxed, calm individual. Anyone can become deficient in GABA, but those who naturally make more of it may feel really off-kilter.

> *Main characteristics of GABA-natured individuals:*
>
> - *Sensible*
> - *Usually on time*
> - *Not prone to mood fluctuations*
> - *Reliable*
> - *Calm under pressure*
> - *Nurturing*
>
> *Foods to enrich GABA:* *Eggs, grains, walnuts, hard cheeses, raw organic spinach, wild fish, fava beans, lentils, and other beans*

Acetylcholine: The Fast-Thinking Neurotransmitter

Another neurotransmitter is acetylcholine, which is also predominantly produced in the brain. Acetylcholine helps with the conduction of nerve impulses and the speed with which neuron signals travel through the brain. If you are an acetylcholine-natured individual, you are probably a fast thinker, and you may be better at multitasking than others, as the nerve impulses in your brain may travel at a faster rate. Acetylcholine-natured individuals are often described as "quick on their feet" and are usually out-of-the-box thinkers with a creative streak. They are also very sensory-oriented individuals and can sometimes rely on their senses more than others.

One of the precursor molecules that helps to make acetylcholine is a fatty molecule called choline. While our body can make a small amount of choline, the majority of it comes from food. The lipid or fatty molecule in choline helps support the cell membranes of our nerve cells. Not eating enough choline, which is present in foods rich in healthy fats such as wild salmon, avocados, shiitake mushrooms, and nuts, can lead to a deficiency in the production of acetylcholine. Acetylcholine deficiencies can trigger brain fog, memory issues, or sluggishness. Acetylcholine-natured people may have more pronounced symptoms and feel like their brains aren't functioning properly if they become deficient.

> ***Main characteristics of acetylcholine-natured individuals:***
>
> * *Quick thinkers—Rely more on their senses*
> * *Fast in most tasks*
> * *Sometimes try to do too much at once*
> * *Highly creative and spontaneous*
> * *Can be impatient*
>
> ***Foods to help increase acetylcholine production:***
> *Fatty fish like salmon, avocados eggs, beans, and mushrooms*

Serotonin: The Adventurous Neurotransmitter

Most individuals are familiar with serotonin, which has been linked to mood, with deficiencies linked to depression. Serotonin is predominantly made in the gut, rather than the brain (approximately 80–90% comes from the gut). However, it certainly has a huge impact on the brain. Serotonin is a mood stabilizer, but it also helps us fall asleep.

Serotonin-natured individuals are usually happy-go-lucky, life-of-the-party types, and tend to be pretty vibrant. If you're serotonin-natured, you're probably always off on adventures and very much in love with life and all the beauty it has to offer. You may spend a lot of time moving around, preferring not to be tied down and you like to try different things.

If you aren't producing enough serotonin, you might find that your mood is affected and you can feel down or possibly even depressed. You might be reluctant to get out and do things, and instead shrink into a routine, preferring the comfort that this offers. You might also find that you struggle to fall asleep at night. If you're a serotonin-natured person, you are again more likely to notice a drastic change if your serotonin levels drop.

Serotonin is produced from an amino acid precursor called tryptophan, which is an essential amino acid. There are 27 amino acids currently known to science, and nine are called essential amino acids, while the others are nonessential. It's important to note that "essential" means your body cannot produce it by itself; thus, it is essential to get these amino acids from food.

Since your body cannot produce tryptophan, you need to eat foods containing it to make more serotonin. Tryptophan is also the precursor for melatonin, which also plays an important role in helping you fall asleep at night. If you are deficient in both serotonin and melatonin, there's a high chance that you will really struggle to fall asleep, meaning that tryptophan is doubly important. Tryptophan is found in foods such as bananas, whole grains, soybeans, nuts, especially walnuts, seeds, and many kinds of meat.

Main characteristics of serotonin-natured individuals:

- *Live in the moment attitude*
- *Optimists*
- *Love to travel and explore*
- *Thrive on change*
- *Life of the party*
- *Always looking for fun opportunities*

Foods to enrich serotonin: Walnuts, bananas, edamame, pumpkin seeds, and most animal proteins

Dopamine: The Excitatory Neurotransmitter

Dopamine is made in both the gut and the brain. It's another neurotransmitter that many people are familiar with because we often talk about the "dopamine high" or "dopamine rush."

Dopamine is an excitatory neurotransmitter that helps you feel enthusiastic or "ready to go." People who are dopamine-natured tend to be highly focused, competitive, and driven, and want to get as much as they can out of life. Interestingly, many successful people who are CEOs or successful in business are dopamine-natured. Having very high levels of dopamine, however, is also common among criminals, so it's possible to have too much of it—but on the whole, we all need dopamine to perform daily tasks.

Dopamine's precursor is tyrosine, which is found in foods such as dark chocolate. As with the other neurotransmitters, if you're not getting enough of this precursor, your dopamine levels may start dropping off, and you'll become deficient. This can make it hard to focus or feel motivated. People with ADHD may have dopamine deficiencies, making it challenging for them to find certain activities rewarding or to focus on them. Interestingly, dopamine surges are also associated with falling in love and the rush that new love offers.

Characteristics of dopamine-natured individuals:

- *Highly competitive*
- *Goal oriented and driven*
- *Strategic thinker and problem solver*
- *Strong willed*
- *Risk taker*

Foods to increase dopamine: *Dark chocolate, green leafy vegetables, coffee, beets, and apples*

Gut–Brain Personalities

You might be wondering now where all of this leaves you. Are you serotonin-natured? GABA-natured? A mix of the two? Naturally dominant in one, but deficient in another due to your diet? Is lack of an important precursor affecting your life and leaving you struggling with mood swings, sleep loss, stress, or something else?

Certainly, having some of these neurotransmitters is important, but it's crucial to recognize that every individual is different, and their dietary requirements can vary enormously. If you're a GABA-dominant individual and you're not eating enough glutamic acid, you're going to feel worse than a serotonin-dominant individual who also isn't eating enough glutamic acid. It makes a big difference, and you should remember that each unique personality may require more specific nutrients than others. This can help you pinpoint precisely what dietary changes might help you feel better.

As an acetylcholine-natured individual, I like to get things done quickly, and my creative streak can sometimes make me an out-of-the-box thinker. By contrast, my husband, who is GABA-dominant, is fairly relaxed and easygoing under pressure. Our dietary needs are very different. While he may opt for foods like cheese or grains, I sometimes crave foods that are rich in fats because those are the ones that will allow me to produce more acetylcholine, fulfilling my natural requirements. Recognizing that while we all need to eat healthy foods, it's important to appreciate our slightly differing needs to achieve overall health and well-being.

I would like to take a moment here to share a story about a patient who was once part of my weight loss program. When her mental health was suboptimal, she would sometimes binge on foods that had brought her short-term comfort as a means of coping with her emotions. She then started creating a daily log of her moods in a journal, and noticed a correlation between unhealthy eating and low mood. Conversely, she found her mood was elevated once she had gotten back on track and started eating well again. She noted that foods like yogurt with sliced bananas and walnuts made her feel uplifted, sometimes in as little as 2–3 days. She started incorporating these foods into her eating plan on a regular basis. What she didn't realize was that she was actually part of her own science experiment because yogurt is rich in Lactobacillus and Bifidobacterium, and bananas and walnuts are both rich in the amino acid tryptophan. All helped her make more serotonin.

Things to Remember

- **GABA is the relaxing neurotransmitter** and GABA-dominant individuals tend to be calm and handle stress well. To ensure your body is producing enough GABA, try to eat fish, nuts, eggs, cheeses, beans, especially soy and fava beans, lentils, whole grains, sunflower seeds, and cocoa.

- **Acetylcholine is the speed neurotransmitter** and acetylcholine-dominant individuals are often creative, good at multitasking, and can think on their feet. To ensure your body is producing enough acetylcholine, try to eat nuts, avocados, wild salmon, eggs, and beans, such as soybeans and kidney beans, as well as chicken, broccoli, brussels sprouts, and shiitake mushrooms.

- **Serotonin is the happy,** adventurous neurotransmitter and serotonin-dominant individuals are vibrant and life-loving. To ensure your body is producing enough serotonin, try to eat bananas, whole grains, nuts and seeds, tofu, fermented foods, spinach, and eggs.

- **Dopamine is the excitatory neurotransmitter** and dopamine-dominant individuals are go-getters who are highly driven and always achieving. To ensure your body is producing enough dopamine, try to eat dark chocolate, almonds, apples, beets, coffee, bananas, and avocados.

- **Production of each neurotransmitter** relies on different precursors, so what you eat is very important in determining how much of each neurotransmitter you make. A varied diet can help you produce a balanced amount of all the neurotransmitters.

- **Every individual has different needs,** meaning your diet should be tailored to your needs.

- **You can access Dr. Braverman's assessment** online if you want to dig deeper into your neurotransmitter dominances and deficiencies.

CHAPTER 10

The Gut–Skin Connection

Your Gut Is Itching to Heal

Like the gut–brain axis, the gut–skin axis is a bidirectional communication network that exists between the gut and the skin.

Gut Health and Common Skin Conditions: From Acne to Eczema, Psoriasis, and Skin Aging

Just as gut inflammation can predispose you to systemic inflammation, it can also cause problems in the skin. Increased gut lining permeability can allow unwanted substances to pass into the bloodstream. Substances can also directly come into contact with the skin from the outside.

Acne and the Gut

Acne has quite a few causes. Gut dysbiosis, hormonal imbalances, or over productive sebaceous glands can precipitate acne. Several studies have already highlighted the fact that hormonal imbalances may trigger acne, but gut bacteria can also influence hormones, affecting this balance.

An enzyme called beta-glucuronidase is produced by certain unhealthy gut microbes. This enzyme breaks down estrogen in the gut, allowing it to be reabsorbed in the bloodstream. In turn, this can increase the amount of estrogen circulating through the body, which may exacerbate acne, and other skin conditions related to estrogen dominance.

There is also a strong inhibitory link between acne and plant-based foods containing **lignans**, mostly found in legumes, seeds, and nuts. A lot of people associate "raging hormones" with teenagers, and that's because there's an increased production of androgens and a surge of hormones flooding the body. Eating foods containing lignans can stabilize these rapid conversions in both estrogen and testosterone, which can also help with acne.

Psoriasis and the Gut

Psoriasis is an autoimmune condition that can also be affected by gut health. We've already seen how autoimmune conditions are linked to leaky gut and faulty immune system activation. Psoriasis is a T-cell-mediated disease. As you may recall in earlier chapters, your body begins producing T cells in response to the "foreign" substances released from the gut. In this case, your skin responds to the inflammation by thickening the epidermis. Sometimes, this thickening extends into the dermis (the outside layer of the skin). The thickening is supposed to be a protective mechanism from the body in an attempt to prevent damage to the skin's barrier, but instead, it results in conditions like psoriasis.

Possible mechanism? Psoriasis, either from a leaky gut or an external skin trigger, causes your immune system to panic, releasing T cells in response. The T cells are intended to fight foreign invaders, help mobilize cytokines, and activate your immune system.

Psoriasis flare-ups linked to dysbiosis are evidenced by higher blood levels of certain toxic biomarkers called lipopolysaccharides (LPS). Remember, LPS toxins are the toxins released by harmful bacteria in the gut. Levels have been shown to decrease once psoriasis flare-ups are under control.

There's also a higher presence of a bacteria called Firmicutes, which in small ratios is not bad but tends to be problematic when found in high ratios. There's a clear correlation between elevated Firmicutes levels, elevated biomarkers, and psoriasis flare-ups.

Eczema and the Gut

Eczema is a common condition and one that I suffered from up until my early 20s. Eczema causes patches of skin to become inflamed, itchy, and rough. Again, studies have shown differences in gut microbiota composition in people with this condition compared to those without it.

It may not be a coincidence that my eczema markedly improved after I lost the remainder of my weight in my early 20s. Not surprisingly, gut dysbiosis is suspected to play a role in eczema flare-ups due to gut dysbiosis, triggering an immune reaction. Certain viral or bacterial infections can also trigger a breakdown in the gut lining by releasing toxic substances. The inflammation causes a similar mechanism of thickening of the skin, along with excessive release of histamine, leading to inflamed, itchy skin.

Various medications such as antibiotics and laxatives as well as vitamin D deficiency have also been linked to eczema. Studies looking at the gut bacteria of patients with eczema, also found lower levels of Bifidobacterium and Akkermansia. Remember that these two beneficial microbes are much lower in patients who are overweight, who also happen to be 1.5 times more likely to suffer from eczema. Coincidentally, I recently did a gut analysis and my Bifidobacterium and Akkermansia levels were optimal, so the gut microbiome IS capable of changing!

Notice a major theme of Bifidobacterium deficiency affecting everything?

The Impact of Gut Dysbiosis on Skin Aging

It's quite likely that there's also a link between the health of your gut and the speed with which your skin ages. Short-chain fatty acids, such as butyrate, propionate, and acetate, work to improve your skin barrier function and maintain your skin hydration. This improves your overall skin health. If you don't have enough short-chain fatty acids, you're more likely to suffer from skin dryness, reduced elasticity, and other signs of aging.

Glycation is a common factor involved in the premature aging of skin. This term refers to a sugar (such as glucose or fructose) attaching to another molecule, such as the skin's elastin or collagen proteins. When sugar molecules weigh down these proteins, your skin becomes more rigid and loses some structural support, causing sagging and wrinkles.

Real-World Case Study

I once had a patient who developed a severe rash all over her body. She already had pre-existing eczema, but noticed it had become worse just prior to seeing me. The itching was so severe that she had started bleeding from all the scratching, and her eczema had spread to her entire body. She had seen a dermatologist, but the topical steroid creams prescribed were not working. She was also experiencing gut issues like constipation and bloating. We first looked at her gut and found elevated Firmicutes/Bacteroidetes ratios in her gut, but she also mentioned that she had just gotten over a strep infection and had received a long course of antibiotics.

We decided to do a rehaul of her diet and I put her on some anti-inflammatory, gut-healing foods, such as bone broth and organic protein-rich foods, and incorporated a healthy plant-based protocol of foods she could tolerate. I minimized refined carbs and removed all processed foods from her diet for 30 days. We also looked at what she was putting on her skin and removed all creams. Within 2 weeks, her eczema had started to improve and within 30 days, it was gone.

Another patient of mine—an 18-year-old bodybuilder, started taking whey protein in addition to a high-fat, high-protein diet, in an effort to bulk up his muscles. He started developing terrible acne as a result. I explained to him that eating only high-protein, high-fat foods along with whey protein affected his hormones and induced acne. He stopped the whey protein and added some antioxidant-rich, plant-based foods to his regimen. Not only did his acne clear up, but he also developed a lean, muscular physique—minus the acne. Many body builders use whey protein, and it's okay occasionally, but it contains an amino acid called leucine, which, in large doses, can trigger acne or eczema.

Things to Remember

- **There is a bidirectional communication network** that exists between our gut and skin, known as the gut–skin axis.
- **Gut dysbiosis has been linked to several common skin conditions,** including acne, eczema, and psoriasis.
- **Gut dysbiosis could potentially influence** the process of skin aging.
- **Avoid foods** such as processed meat, high-sugar treats, and fried food such as chicken nuggets and fries to decrease the glycation process.
- **Eat more foods** like antioxidant-rich fruits and vegetables, including broccoli, asparagus, leafy greens, kimchi, leeks, onions, and other fiber-rich and fermented foods to support a healthy gut microbiome. This will help stabilize the ratio of Firmicutes/Bacteroides.
- **Avoid unnecessary use of antibiotics,** which can disrupt the balance of the gut microbiome.

- **Some foods that are rich in lignans can help with acne and include** onions, garlic, pumpkin and sesame seeds, flaxseeds, apricots, brussels sprouts, and blueberries.
- **Decrease estrogen dominance** by maintaining a healthy BMI, especially in postmenopause.

CHAPTER 11

Prebiotics and Probiotics
The Role in Gut Health

In this chapter, we will be reviewing how prebiotics and probiotics are essential for a healthy, balanced diet. We have already touched upon them in previous chapters, but now it's time to understand why and how they work. Probiotics are beneficial live microorganisms, while prebiotics are dietary fibers that nourish these organisms in the gut.

Summarizing Prebiotic and Probiotic Food Sources

Prebiotics are the fuel for your beneficial gut bacteria; they're what your gut bacteria feed on. They occur naturally in high-fiber foods.

We've identified a few types of plant-based foods that our gut friends like to feed on.

- **Sources of inulin fiber** such as onions, garlic, leeks, asparagus, chicory root, and artichokes. Inulin is a favorite food for most beneficial bacteria. They will feed on it, digest it, and make postbiotics with it, and then the rest is passed out of the body as waste. Strains like Bifidobacterium and Lactobacillus are both heavily dependent on getting enough inulin to survive and grow.

- **Root and tuber fibers** such as those found in parsnips, potatoes, carrots, beets, taro, and turnips.
- **Resistant starch** fibers include beans, sweet potatoes, barley, and bananas. Foods that your upper gastrointestinal tract is not good at digesting tend to be the best for providing prebiotics. If they aren't digested early in the process, they reach the colon, and here, the beneficial organisms can feed on them, ferment them, and grow stronger.
- **Fruit-based fibers** such as oranges, apples, and blueberries are also loved by our beneficial microbes. Think of them as dessert for the little guys. They are also rich in important **antioxidants** that we need for certain important vitamins such as vitamin C.

Probiotics are beneficial bacteria that offer numerous health benefits when they are eaten in the right amounts. They occur naturally in various foods, particularly those that have been fermented.

- **Miso, kimchi, pickled foods, sauerkraut, kefir, yogurt, tempeh**, and certain kinds of **aged cheeses**, including Gouda, and cheddar are good examples of this. It is important to be somewhat cautious of cheeses; they contain beneficial microbes and important probiotics but are also high in saturated fats like omega-6. Small quantities of omega-6 are okay, but consuming too much may have harmful effects on the body. Kefir and yogurt are often better sources of probiotics as they are lower in saturated fats.

Fermented foods offer a rich source of bacteria, which helps to diversify and replenish your gut microbiota. They also aid in the digestion and absorption of nutrients, and influence the overall health of your gut microbiome. Consuming them regularly helps the microbiome stay strong.

How to Choose the Right Probiotic Supplement

It is important to remember that supplements are exactly what they are noted to be–"supplements" to a healthy diet. As I have mentioned in previous chapters, my philosophy on probiotics is that they are good to add to a healthy diet, but you can't probiotic your way out of an unhealthy gut. There are three key things to look for when choosing a probiotic:

- The first of these is *strain specificity*. Different strains of probiotics offer different health benefits. Some strains of Bifidobacterium and Lactobacillus are known to support gut health and regulate bowel movements. It's therefore important to choose supplements with strains that are most likely to address your specific health conditions. Additionally, different beneficial probiotic strains often work in symbiotic ways, so it's often best to find multistrain probiotics (although temporary use of single-strain probiotics may be useful when treating a specific gut issue). Relying on just a supplement instead of food can also decrease your gut diversity since you're getting the same strains in the probiotic instead of those from different foods. This is why probiotics should not be taken consistently, to encourage diversity of the gut from other sources.

- You also need to look at the **CFU count**. This stands for colony-forming unit, which indicates how many live microbes are in the supplement. You need to pay attention to the end-of-shelf-life CFU. It doesn't matter what the CFU is when the product is produced because the manufacturers can easily add a lot of probiotics at this point, but what matters is how many there are when it has been sitting on a shelf for a long time.

Many probiotics sit at room temperature, which may kill some strains, especially if they remain there for a long time. Refrigerated products may be better, as this will help to keep the probiotics alive longer. That's not to say there are no good room-temperature probiotics, but often, some of the bacteria will be lost during transportation and storage, so if you choose a nonrefrigerated kind, look for ones that are heat-resistant and have a higher CFU count (minimum 30 billion) so you ensure as many as possible will survive the stomach acid during passage to your intestines.

- *Quality* of the probiotic will also make a difference. Some probiotics have been used in clinical studies and while these may cost a bit more, they are what we call medical grade and have been shown to produce the desired effects in the studies.

Taking the three major factors—strain specificity, CFU count, and quality of the product—into account when you choose a probiotic will make it much easier to choose one that is right for you. I still prefer food as the best source of probiotics, but when that is not always possible, it's worth understanding supplements.

A further consideration is when you take your probiotic supplement. You generally want to take a probiotic on an empty stomach. This is because your stomach produces more acid when you eat, which may destroy some probiotics before they pass into the intestines. You should therefore aim to take a probiotic first thing in the morning or just before you go to sleep.

Do not take an antibiotic and probiotic simultaneously if you are taking an antibiotic. Bear in mind that the antibiotics' job is to kill harmful microbes—so if you combine the two, the antibiotics may simply kill off some of the beneficial bacteria. You should therefore take them approximately 3 or 4 hours apart if possible.

The Role of Synbiotics in Gut Health

There are also products called **synbiotics**, which are both pre and probiotics together. They are designed to establish and improve the survival of beneficial live bacteria in the gut. These usually incorporate both plant-based fibers and fermented foods, so you get "the best of both worlds." They provide the body with beneficial bacteria and nourishment to support them.

Synbiotics can be found naturally in foods like pickles—a cucumber contains fiber, but it has been fermented too, so you also get the probiotic element. An added bonus in pickles is that the liquid brine has been shown to help with muscle cramps, sometimes instantaneously!

Some studies have shown that the acidic nature of the brine can inhibit the nerve impulses that cause muscle cramps and many professional athletes swear by this. There's also kimchi, which contains fiber from the cabbage and beneficial bacteria from the fermentation process. It's interesting to note that certain cultures, like Egyptians and Greeks, have long histories of fermentation of many different kinds of foods, including turnips and radishes. With their food preservation techniques, our ancestors probably enjoyed much better health than we do, considering they had limited access to healthcare.

Things to Remember

- **Consume a variety of prebiotics fibers for a more diverse gut.**
- **Prebiotics, probiotics, and synbiotics (postbiotics that are both prebiotics and probiotics)** play crucial roles in maintaining a healthy gut microbiome.
- **Probiotic supplements** should be used as just that—supplements, and not solely relied upon for improved gut health.

CHAPTER 12

Environment and Social Connections
How They Affect Your Health

Your gut is always responding to your surroundings, from the air you breathe to the food you eat; everything affects your gut. In this chapter, we're going to explore how the environment and social connections affect you and what you can do about it.

Environmental Toxins and Gut Health

Whether it's a chemical in a cleaning product, a pesticide in your food, or heavy metals in your drinking water, chronic exposure to certain chemicals can cause dysbiosis in the gut.

Artificial food coloring, such as **red number 40**, is found in many products, including popular candies, cereals, and countless other products. Several studies have revealed that this coloring can destroy beneficial bacteria in the gut. It has also been shown to worsen the symptoms of ADHD. It is either banned in some European countries or requires labeling, stating that it has adverse effects on activity and attention in children. It has also been shown to worsen symptoms of inflammatory bowel disease. If you've been to Europe, you may have noticed that the red-colored candies don't quite have the same vibrancy that candies in the United States have. Now you know why.

Artificial sweeteners, like **sucralose** and **aspartame**, have also been shown to affect the gut. Some studies have even shown that sucralose can affect a person's DNA. Aspartame is broken down in the body into two chemicals called aspartic acid and phenylalanine, both of which have been shown to affect the central nervous system. In mice, breaking down sucralose and aspartame has been shown to increase anxiety symptoms.

Another environmental toxin is **fluoride**, and this is difficult to avoid exposure to. In the 1950s, fluoride was given to individuals because it was thought that it could strengthen teeth. This is still the case in many countries today, and fluoride is frequently added to the water. While fluoride may strengthen the tooth enamel and reduce your risk of cavities, it has also been shown to negatively affect the gut. Speaking of teeth and good oral hygiene, one simple way to improve your microbiome's health is to brush your teeth just before sleeping. The microbiome starts in the mouth, and many harmful bacteria produce plaque, which can travel through our blood vessels and cause inflammation. Studies have shown that this can markedly increase the risk of heart disease. Obviously, brushing in the morning is important too, but at night, salivary glands are less effective at clearing plaque.

Another environmental toxin to be aware of is **glyphosate**, a pesticide used to kill weeds growing in many crops. Glyphosate has been identified as a carcinogen and has also been shown to disrupt the microbiome and destroy beneficial organisms in the gut. To avoid glyphosate, you may want to choose organic foods when possible.

A list of gut disruptors is not complete without mentioning **seed oils**. These oils are highly processed and have been shown to increase inflammation in the gut, leading to systemic inflammation. Some popular seed oils you'll want to avoid are rapeseed oil, palm oil, canola oil, soybean oil, sunflower oil, corn oil, rice bran oil, and margarine. Oils that might be better choices are olive oil and avocado oil, as well as butter and ghee.

CHEAT SHEET
OF HEALTHY OILS

HEALTHY OILS	VS.	UNHEALTHY OILS
Olive Oil – Extra Virgin– Low smoke point. Perfect for dressings and drizzles. **Regular Olive Oil–**Medium smoke point. More suitable for roasting, grilling, and sautéing.		Canola oil
Macadamia Nut Oil–High smoke point. Ideal for stir fry and sautéd dishes.		Corn oil
Avocado Oil–High smoke point. Great for sautéing, roasting, searing, grilling, and drizzles.		Soybean oil
Walnut Oil–Low smoke point. Best for salad dressings and drizzles, not as a frying oil.		Peanut oil
Grass-Fed Ghee–High smoke point. Excellent as a sauteing and baking oil. Has a great buttery taste.		Sunflower-Safflower oil
Grass-Fed Butter–Low smoke point. Best used in baking or spreads, not in frying, sautéing, and grilling.		Margarine

@doctorchristineb

CHEAT SHEET OF HEALTHY SWEETENERS

VS.

HEALTHY SWEETENERS

- **Honey:** Raw, organic and Manuka honey contain antioxidants and have antimicrobial properties.
- **Monk fruit:** Sweeter than sugar, with no calories and no effect on blood sugar levels.
- **Stevia:** A natural sweetener with zero calories, but use in small amounts.
- **Fruits:** Natural sweetness, fiber, vitamins, and minerals.
- **Maple syrup:** Minerals and antioxidants.

UNHEALTHY SWEETENERS

- Aspartame
- Sucralose
- Saccharin
- Acesulfame potassium
- Sorbitol
- Xylitol
- Erythritol
- Advantame
- High-fructose corn syrup

@doctorchristineb   **Christine Bishara MD**

Whenever you choose an oil, it's important to be aware of the oil's smoke point, which refers to how much heat you can use when cooking with it. If you heat the oil above its smoke point, it will not only taste bad, but it can become carcinogenic. Avocado oil has a smoke point of around 520°F, so it's one of the best options if you're cooking at high temperatures.

Olive oil has a lower smoke point, so while it's healthy, you shouldn't cook with it at very high temperatures. That's particularly true for extra virgin olive oil with a smoke point of around 410°F and butter which has a smoke point of 350°F. Ghee is another great option with a smoke point of 480°F.

Another environmental toxin to be aware of is *bisphenol A*, one of the **BPAs**. These are found in certain kinds of plastics, including some plastic containers that are marked as food-safe. Plastic water bottles may also include it, although both are becoming less common as awareness of BPA and its dangers has risen. More stable plastics tend to be used now, but you should be careful and always check what the plastic container says on its base. There will usually be a number ranging from 1 to 7 on the bottom of any plastic bottle or cup. This number, the Resin Identification Code indicates how stable the plastic is. The higher the number, the more stable the plastic and its ability to withstand temperature changes.

If you've used disposable spring water bottles, you'll probably be aware that these are very flimsy and don't stand up to much use. They usually have a number 1 Resin ID. Refilling them puts additional "stress" on the plastic which it wasn't designed to withstand thus, increasing the possibility of leakage of the plastic into your drink. The same goes for freezing water bottles. Some people love to put their water bottles in the freezer to enjoy a chilled beverage, but disposable water bottles aren't designed to withstand this and may start to leach chemicals into the water when expanded. If you want to freeze or heat the container, make sure you choose one with a high number, or use nonplastic containers instead.

Another source of exposure to toxins is clothing made with synthetic dyes and other toxic chemicals. This is sometimes termed "fast fashion," and not only are these harmful toxins present in the clothing, but many factories in Asia and the surrounding area release contaminated wastewater into water supplies. One simple step to decrease your exposure is to wash all clothing before it is worn.

Heavy metals and certain over-the-counter medications are also worth being mindful of. *Mercury* is a heavy metal sometimes found in fish, such as swordfish and tuna.

Some medications, such as senna laxatives, can disrupt the gut's microbiome and lead to a condition called lazy colon or melanosis coli—a medical term for abnormal discoloration of the gut lining seen in colonoscopies of patients who have been on senna for prolonged periods. *Senna* stimulates the gut to eliminate waste, but if your gut and intestines become tolerant to the effects of senna, they will stop working independently. The peristaltic muscle contractions that help the muscles contract properly will not be as effective, leading to rebound chronic constipation.

Tips for Reducing Exposure to Environmental Toxins

The idea that there are many dangers around you in everyday life might feel a bit overwhelming, but there's a lot you can do. The body is capable of handling some insults, but taking small incremental measures can help reduce your exposure. I still sometimes accidentally forget to read a label and find that a product contains a seed oil or artificial sweetener, but I have become more aware and more vigilant.

The EWG is an organization that publishes a list of the fruits and vegetables with the highest and lowest toxins annually. The most toxic are called the Dirty Dozen and the least toxic are called The Clean Fifteen. You should try to buy organic from the foods on the Dirty Dozen List. The list changes annually, but many foods are always on the list.

The most common Dirty Dozen foods that make the list almost every year include:

- Strawberries
- Spinach
- Kale, collars, mustard greens
- Peaches
- Pears
- Nectarines
- Apples
- Grapes
- Bell and hot peppers
- Cherries
- Blueberries
- Green beans

These fruits and vegetables are most likely to contain high levels of pesticides. If you don't have options to buy organic, soak the fruit/vegetable in water with a tablespoon of baking soda for 15 minutes. Studies have shown that baking soda will help pull out most pesticides, and then you can rinse the vegetable and pat it dry. This isn't a foolproof method, but it does help.

The most common foods on the Clean Fifteen list are:

- Avocados
- Sweetcorn

- Pineapples
- Onions
- Papayas
- Sweet peas
- Asparagus
- Honeydew melons
- Kiwis
- Cabbages
- Mushrooms
- Mangoes
- Sweet potatoes
- Watermelons
- Carrots

It may still be worth buying organic if you are able to, but these foods should be safer to eat if you don't have access to organic ones.

You can check out these lists on EWG.ORG as they get updated yearly. You can also download the app to have a handy guide when you go shopping. Use it to guide your food choices.

Often, when you're shopping for fruits and vegetables in the United States, you'll also note that they have stickers with different numbers on them. They might look meaningless at first, but each number tells you something about how the vegetable was grown. You can use these to be more grocery-savvy.

If you see a four-digit code, that means it has been "conventionally raised," which generally means it was grown with pesticides in poor soil. If you see a five-digit code starting with a 9, the food is organic. Some people remember this using the "nine-is-fine" mantra. If the code is five digits but starts with an 8, it has been genetically modified " I hate 8." These numbers change periodically, so be mindful and do your homework.

If you have the option, buying locally at a farmer's market is often an excellent idea. You may even be able to talk to the farmer about how they grow their food, where their farm is, etc. It's important to remember that being certified as organic by the USDA involves quite a process, and some small farmers may choose not to do this for cost reasons—but might still grow food organically. This could also be a good option.

The Influence of Social Factors on Gut Health: What We Can Learn from "The Roseto Effect"

Social factors have a profound impact on your health, including your gut health. Chronic stress can disrupt the balance of your gut microbiome and compromise the function of the gut barrier.

These gut disruptions can also prevent the body from producing the neurotransmitters it needs to maintain a good mood. They can also have an impact on sleep and cognitive functioning.

One example of the power of social connections on our health is from a study from the 1960s. You may have heard of the Roseto Effect before, but if you haven't, it refers to a study done in a small town in Roseto, Pennsylvania. This study offers a fascinating example of why diet isn't everything when it comes to determining your health and why social connections make a huge difference too.

If you're not familiar with it, the town of Roseto, Pennsylvania caused researchers a great deal of confusion in the 1960s. Many of the townspeople smoked and ate a diet high in fat, albeit, meals were made from fresh ingredients. Despite these risk factors, they had significantly lower rates of heart disease and tended to live longer than the national average. Researchers were baffled and spent some time studying what was affording the community members this extra protection.

They eventually pinpointed what made Roseto different: the families who lived there had very strong social connections and close-knit communities. Many living in the community were Italian immigrants who frequently ate together and enjoyed many social activities with one another.

Another factor that researchers believe contributed to this longevity was that many of the households had multiple generations living within them, consisting of grandparents living with their children and grandchildren. The grandparents tended to be very involved in the grandchildren's lives, keeping them socially active and connected, elevating their overall health. Additionally, grandchildren were also highly involved in their grandparents' lives, strengthening their social connections with adults and providing a strong support network.

This may echo how people tended to live in the past, where many family members of varied ages would live in one home, rather than just parents and children. There wasn't as much social isolation, and people participated in more social activities—something we have lost in most nuclear families today.

The Roseto Effect has helped us understand that while diet is important, having a close-knit community and a strong social network can also make an enormous difference in our health and longevity. We could all stand to learn a lot from Roseto.

Other Factors

The Importance of Being Outdoors

The value of being outdoors should not be underestimated either; there is enormous benefit to your overall health and well-being, but also specifically to your gut health. The idea of "forest therapy" may sound a little unusual, but it has been shown that trees and many other plants produce compounds that are useful to humans when we breathe them in. Plenty of plants emit antimicrobial and insecticidal compounds, collectively called phytoncides (literally meaning "plant" and "kill").

These compounds have been shown to be beneficial when we breathe them in; they can even prompt an anti-inflammatory effect and may reduce stress and cortisol levels. Furthermore, phytoncides increase the activity of natural killer cells—the white blood cells that are responsible for protecting your body against illnesses.

Not everybody finds it easy to spend time in nature, but the rewards of doing so can be almost limitless, and this is a key part of protecting yourself and promoting good gut health.

Iodine and Its Effect

It is also worth being aware of the importance of iodine for overall health, especially gut, thyroid, and breast health. One hundred years ago, iodine deficiency was uncommon in the United States or most seaside areas (although it might have been seen elsewhere). This is because iodine was added in minuscule amounts to table salt, so most people were getting adequate iodine either from food or from bathing in the ocean, which is rich in iodine. Now, many people restrict salt or use noniodized salts such as Himalayan salt, contributing to an iodine deficiency crisis.

Some groups at *higher risk* for iodine deficiency include pregnant women and vegans. Those living in areas with low levels of iodine in the soil or not near the ocean are also at risk.

Good *sources* of *iodine* include:

- Seaweed (such as kelp, nori, kombu, and wakame)
- Fish and other seafood
- Dairy products
- Eggs
- Iodized salt

Iodine deficiency has been implicated in an increased risk of breast cancer, thyroid conditions, and thyroid cancer. Iodine is essential for thyroid hormone synthesis and helps reduce estrogen sensitivity in the breasts as well. The best way to include iodine in your diet is through iodine-rich foods, including seaweed, eggs, beef liver, chicken, fish, and shellfish. Iodized salt can be added if needed.

Self-medicating with oral iodine should NOT be undertaken as it could have a negative impact on your thyroid. Always check with your doctor before starting iodine, especially if you have a thyroid condition.

Things to Remember

- **Exposure to environmental toxins** can disrupt the gut microbiome, affecting your overall health.
- **Strong social bonds improve your overall health,** including your gut health.
- **Avoid Seed oils, artificial dyes, and artificial sweeteners** by reading read labels carefully.
- **Wash all new clothing** before you wear them.
- **Stay updated with the list of harmful foods and products** on the EWG website EWG.ORG.
- **Ensure adequate iodine intake** through food.
- **Spend time outdoors** often for the benefits of modest sun exposure and inhalation of beneficial phytoncides.
- **Choose helpful sweeteners,** such as honey, monk fruit, stevia (in small quantities), fruits, and maple syrup.
- **Avoid unhealthy sweeteners** such as aspartame, sucralose, saccharin, acesulfame potassium, sorbitol, xylitol, erythritol, advantame, and high-fructose corn syrup.

CHAPTER 13

Personalized Gut Health

We Are All the Same, Yet We Are All Different

In this chapter, we're going to look at genetic and lifestyle differences that can impact your gut health. We already know that while there are some generalizations to be made, our gut microbiome is unique to each of us, and what's ideal for one person may be less for another. That uniqueness has made it somewhat difficult to fully understand gut health. However, there are a few organisms that have definitely been identified as beneficial. We can also identify certain markers that may signify if an individual is at risk of developing certain conditions in the future.

The Human Microbiome Project

The Human Microbiome Project was an intensive endeavor conducted by the National Institute of Health, unveiling the microbiome's incredible diversity. This study demonstrated that even healthy individuals differ remarkably in the composition of their microbiota and that our guts are highly individualized.

This project studied the microbiome of individuals in many nations worldwide and found that industrialized nations aren't doing very well when it comes to gut diversity. The project also looked at an interesting African tribe, called the Hadza tribe. This is one of the few remaining hunter–gatherer tribes. They eat only what they catch and only seasonal fruits and vegetables from their local environment. Their diets change with the seasons. They have a very low incidence of heart disease and diabetes despite lacking access to medical care or healthcare facilities. Their gut microbiomes were found to be among the most diverse in the world.

COVID-19 provided a much-needed wake-up call regarding our vulnerability to diseases, but few studies have fully recognized just how important health and lifestyle are as preventive factors. One study that has looked at this in more detail was completed in 2016 and explored the correlation between Bifidobacterium levels, aging, and disease resistance: "evidence is accumulating which shows beneficial effects of supplementation with Bifidobacteria for the improvement of human health conditions ranging from protection against infection to different extra- and intra-intestinal positive effects."

I also explored this relationship in my 2020 review study, specifically in relation to the body's ability to defend against COVID-19–*Could Certain Strains of Gut Bacteria Play a Role in the Prevention and Potential Treatment of COVID-19 Infections?*

Many different factors, including genetics, diet, lifestyle, and the environment, shape the gut's uniqueness. Individual differences significantly affect our susceptibility to certain diseases, the ways in which we respond to different treatments, and our mood and behavior. Understanding these differences is the first step in personalized gut health.

Identifying Areas for Improvement in Your Gut Health

Understanding how your gut is currently functioning is a crucial first step. Consider keeping a food and mood diary and try to make a correlation between the things you eat and the way you feel—physically and mentally. This can provide insights into what's going on. Digestive symptoms such as bloating, heartburn, constipation, acne, diarrhea, etc. can all signify gut dysbiosis.

If you have the resources, you could consider getting a gut microbiome analysis and consulting with a healthcare professional who understands the importance of gut health.

Recognizing Personal Genetic Differences

Because everyone is so different, it's important to think about your gut on a personal level. It's also worth bearing in mind that some of the differences between us may come down to our genetics and the things our ancestors ate, affecting what our bodies have adapted to eating. If you are of Asian or African descent, for example, you're much more likely to be lactose intolerant than if you are European. Countries with higher temperatures have a higher incidence of lactose intolerance. It's likely that this is because cows raised in a hot climate were more likely to produce milk that became spoiled, making the populations consuming the milk sick. Over time, the body adapted to this by becoming lactose intolerant, leading to reduced consumption of milk. In cold environments, with fewer infected milk products, the body did not need to make this adaptation as frequently.

Another study found that how individuals respond to different types of bread was highly dependent on their gut microbiome, which also relies partially on genetic predispositions. Certain populations tend to have a better tolerance of carbohydrates than others if ancestors ate more carbohydrate-rich foods. They were found to have higher levels of amylase, a salivary enzyme that breaks down carbohydrates. The more you have of this enzyme, the more tolerant you are of carbohydrates.

Looking at what your ancestors ate can tell you what you're more likely to tolerate and what foods may benefit your gut. Eating a diet similar to your ancestors' is more likely to be agreeable to you and beneficial for your gut.

A Very Common Gene Defect You Need to Know About

Other important genetic factors include a common gene defect called the **MTHFR gene** mutation. This defect has been reported in over one-third of the population and is a crucial part of a DNA repair process called **methylation**. Methylation is a chemical process that helps stabilize your DNA; it's a biochemical pathway that our bodies activate more than a million times daily. MTHFR is necessary for the creation, maintenance, and repair of DNA, and it also helps with the detoxification process—but if the gene is mutated, these tasks may not be completed as smoothly. This can affect your ability to filter out environmental toxins, absorb nutrients, and produce dopamine.

The significance of MTHFR gene mutation has only been recently recognized, and it has been linked with many health conditions, including ADHD, Alzheimer's disease, cardiovascular diseases, infertility, birth defects, mental health problems, and more. While 30–40% of individuals have a defect in the MTHFR gene, severity can vary. The impact on the DNA has a multitude of symptoms, and being aware of the defect is key so that you can take steps to mitigate its impact on you. It's possible to get tested for the MTHFR gene defect through a blood test, and treatments may include taking methylated vitamin B12, practicing intermittent fasting, minimizing alcohol intake, and eating a prebiotic and probiotic-rich diet to increase your body's production of butyrate, which helps with the detoxification pathways that are affected by methylation.

Understanding whether you have the MTHFR gene defect is another key part of tailoring your gut health journey to your specific needs and ensuring your body gets what it needs despite the defect. This is just one aspect of personalizing your approach to a healthy gut, but it is a key one, and it is usually done with a simple saliva or blood test.

In my practice, I have repeatedly found that many of these factors play a role in personalized recommendations to improve overall health, weight loss, and mental well-being.

Finding the Motivation to Maintain Gut Health

One of the best ways to get motivated to change your gut health is to remember all the benefits that you stand to gain. Tracking and keeping journals on your progress can help you stay the course. I've seen over and over with those who are successful that a large part of the process is in building habits, being consistent in lifestyle decisions, and planning and journaling.

Another great strategy is connecting with others following a similar journey. This creates a sense of community and support, and could even help you tap into the Roseto Effect if you find a strong sense of connection. An added bonus is that your gut microbiome is impacted by the people you spend time with. That might sound astonishing, but our microbiomes are shared with those we spend the most time with—so if you're trying to lose weight, spending time with thin individuals and eating meals with them could positively impact your microbiome. Thin individuals have adequate Bifidobacterium and Akkermansia levels, and believe it or not, your microbiome may begin to mimic theirs, helping you lose weight too.

Things to Remember

- **Gut health is highly individualized** and understanding individual differences is key to personalized gut health.
- **Recognizing your current gut health status and setting personalized goals** can help tailor your gut health plan.
- **Tracking your progress** and adjusting your plan as needed is crucial in your gut health journey.
- **Staying motivated and overcoming challenges** are important for maintaining gut health in the long run.

CHAPTER 14

The Gut Revolution
Getting Started

Now it's time to implement everything you've learned into a lifestyle habit. These are general guidelines and may need to be tailored to your unique gut–brain personality and dietary needs and restrictions. Remember, you can outsource many things in your life, but you can't outsource your health.

I've outlined the steps in a DO's and DON'Ts list to make it easier to follow:

The Do's

- *Do* **plan your meals**: whether your goal is to improve your gut health or lose weight, two meals and a small snack are sufficient, especially if they come from foods that will satisfy your gut microbes and get those postbiotic satiety signals working.
  To induce this, 70% of your meals should be from a plant-based source. The best way to calculate this would be to think of your plate as a pie chart. Seventy percent of the plate should include a plant-based vegetable or legume and 30% should be an "other."

The other source could be anything you might want to add for that meal, whether it be a small amount of animal protein, or a healthy starch such as some high-fiber whole grain bread or a potato, for example. Animal protein should be either grass-fed or organic. Be sure to include enough protein in your pie ratio, whether that comes from the plant-based source or the "other." Most people do not need to eat three meals. Two meals or two meals and a snack daily is enough. ***Do* get creative** when choosing plant-based foods, aiming for a variety of 30 different types per week. Many of my patients like to make a smoothie as their "snack," and it can be a good way to get several fruit and vegetable servings into one meal. Frozen organic fruits are great because you can always have them on hand and you can experiment with different flavor combinations. Other options to add are fresh spinach, celery, etc. If you eat as suggested with the 70/30 ratio in mind, calorie counting may not be needed, but eating 1300–1600 calories of mostly plant-based food will usually result in weight loss. If your goal is improved gut health, you can incorporate these suggestions and add a third meal.

- ***Do* drink *water*** before each meal and one cup on rising in the morning. You can add lemon or cucumber, which can help awaken your GI system while not overwhelming it in the morning. Room temperature water is best for that first morning cup.

- *Do* **incorporate fermented foods** at least 3–4 times per week. The best-fermented foods are those that are also plant-based, so you're getting both prebiotics and probiotics in one shot.
- *Do* **give your body a time of *fasting*** daily. Fasting does NOT mean starvation. It means restricting the hours that you eat during the day, optimally eating during a 6–8-hour window for weight loss or 8–12 hours for improved gut health. This time of restriction will help your body detoxify, while your gut works on other important functions, other than digestion. It also prevents chronic insulin surges. Intermittent fasting does not mean unlimited calories. Try to do this at least 5 days a week.
- *Do* **get at least 7–8 hours of *sleep* nightly.** Insufficient sleep leads to insulin resistance and elevated cortisol levels, which can lead to appetite instability.
- *Do* **eat as much *organic food* as possible**, especially fruits and vegetables on the "dirty dozen list." These are fruits and vegetables you should never eat unless they are organic. Consult with the EWG website to see updated lists: WWW.EWG.ORG.
- *Do* **rinse all fruits and vegetables**, even organic. If you must eat nonorganic fruit, soak it in a bowl of water with some baking soda for 15 minutes and then rinse. Baking soda has been shown to remove a majority of the pesticides present in food.
- *Do* **wash all clothing and bed sheets** prior to wearing/using, as many contain harsh chemicals and allergens that can be absorbed through the skin.

- *Do* **use these oils:** olive, avocado, coconut, walnut, and macadamia. Butter and ghee are also good. Read labels. Oils to avoid include canola, corn, soybean, peanut, sunflower, safflower, and margarine.
- *Do* **prepare healthy meals** ahead of time. This makes a big difference since you will have a healthy option ready to eat when you're hungry.
- *Do* **include a variety** of vibrant and colorful fruits and vegetables. These foods are rich in powerful antioxidants. Antioxidants are important because they help to stabilize damaging particles in the body called **free radicals**. The more antioxidants you consume, the less free radical damage to cells.

The Don'ts

- *Don't* **eat or drink anything with artificial** sweeteners of any kind. These have endocrine disruptors and will lead to a vicious cycle of gut inflammation, negatively affecting your gut–brain axis and making you hungry.
- *Don't* **start any meal with something sweet**, but instead, eat a fiber-rich or savory food first. This is to avoid dramatic glucose and insulin spikes and instead lead to a more steady rise in your blood glucose levels.
- *Don't* **jump off the bandwagon** just because you have 1 or 2 bad days. REDIRECTION, OPTIMISM, and GRIT are the keys to success, remember that.
- *Don't* **eat farmed fish/seafood of any kind**. Check labels carefully. It should be noted as wild.

- ***Don't* microwave any plastic containers**. Don't freeze or refill plastic water bottles.
- ***Don't* weigh yourself daily**, if your goal is to lose weight. The scale is fickle, and your weight can vary depending on many factors. My recommendation is to weigh 1–2 times per week. To better track your progress, use a measuring tape.

Top Fifty Best Plant-Based Foods
for Your Gut

Artichokes	Kale
Onions	Parsnips
Garlic	Cabbage
Asparagus	Okra
Chicory root	Carrots
Mushrooms	Turnips
Raw Spinach	String beans
Broccoli	Edamame
Brussels sprouts	Watercress
Beets	Arugula
Sweet potatoes	Sprouts
Lentils	Leeks
Black beans	Kidney beans
Cauliflower	Chickpeas
Celery	String beans
Strawberries	Beets
Cranberries	Fennel
Blueberries	Radishes
Blackberries	Dandelion
Apples	Seaweed
Bananas	Watermelon
Oranges	Cantaloupes
Mangoes	Grapefruits
Taro	Peaches
Watercress	Guavas

Nuts and seeds are also great add-ons, but should be in small quantities (less than a handful) as they are high in calories.

Best Nutrient Dense Nuts and Seeds

Walnuts		Pumpkin seeds
Pecans		Basil seeds
Almonds		

Best Probiotic Rich Foods

Kefir	Kombucha
Tempeh	Yogurt
Sauerkraut	Kimchi
Miso	Pickled foods

Before you start your gut health journey, schedule an appointment with your doctor to get some baseline labs, including magnesium and vitamin D levels. I personally also like to add a gut microbiome analysis so I can see what is going on in the gut and what ratios of beneficial/harmful microbes are present along with other inflammatory markers that may be present. Be sure to keep up to date with health screenings like colonoscopies, and others as recommended by your physician. These suggestions are only general guidelines. Each individual is unique and has certain nutritional needs that should be discussed with your doctor.

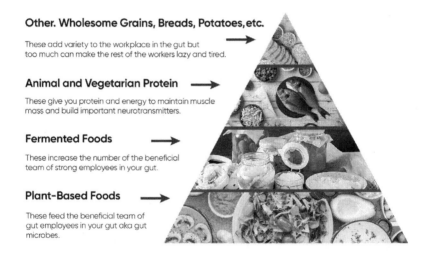

Other. Wholesome Grains, Breads, Potatoes,etc.

These add variety to the workplace in the gut but too much can make the rest of the workers lazy and tired.

Animal and Vegetarian Protein

These give you protein and energy to maintain muscle mass and build important neurotransmitters.

Fermented Foods

These increase the number of the beneficial team of strong employees in your gut.

Plant-Based Foods

These feed the beneficial team of gut employees in your gut aka gut microbes.

CHAPTER 15

The Future of Gut Health
Innovations and Developments

Gut health is a field that we are still learning more about. There is so much we have learned, but there's still much to learn about the trillions of organisms that reside within us and affect our health. Will AI play a role in our gut health? Will there be lasting impacts of COVID-19 affecting our gut?

Innovations in Gut Health Diagnostics

Technological advancements have brought us some phenomenal developments in recent years. These have included next-generation sequencing (NGS), which helps us better study the genetic variation associated with diseases, and metagenomics, which is the study of genetic material from environmental and clinical samples. NGS has transformed how we understand the microbial world of the gut by allowing researchers to accurately identify and catalog the millions of different microorganisms living in the gut. These techniques have allowed us to map the human microbiome, which will guide future healthcare approaches.

There's also a new aspect of diagnostics that evaluates the metabolic byproducts of our microbiome. This field's development has given us a better understanding of microbial activities and how they interact with the host's metabolism. More work is needed, but this is a promising tool for improving gut health in the future.

Other recent advancements include breath testing for many conditions, including small intestinal bacterial overgrowth—a noninvasive method of evaluating a patient's current health safely and comfortably. These methods are the forerunners of much more precise medical techniques, and we anticipate that in-depth, personalized microbial data will soon guide many therapeutic decisions.

Personalized Nutrition for Gut Health

We have thoroughly established just how fundamental the role of diet is in shaping the gut microbiota, but personalized nutrition represents taking this a step further. This is about tailoring dietary interventions based on an individual's unique biological makeup, including their gut microbiome. We now understand that different individuals respond differently to various foods and that a one-size-fits-all approach is not the most effective when it comes to managing gut health.

We have already begun personalizing treatment measures based on each person's unique metabolic makeup and gut microbiome. Of course, most of the research is in its early stages, but it looks very promising. In the future, we might see doctors making use of detailed gut microbiome data to inform healthcare decisions, improve dietary choices, and increase disease prevention. It will be fascinating to see where this goes and what we can learn from it.

The Role of Artificial Intelligence in Gut Health Research

There have been some incredible advancements in gut health diagnostics in recent years and AI in particular will likely play a role in these advancements. It is still in its early stages, but it may be able to offer us incredible medical advancements, potentially revolutionizing the way we predict and diagnose diseases. The gut microbiome is so complex that AI is perfect for analyzing it and drawing conclusions from it. Machine learning algorithms can analyze extensive datasets, uncover patterns, make predictions, and guide personalized interventions. Of course, this could also be detrimental if it's used as a form of bioweapon.

We can now even determine whether you are at risk for a particular condition by looking at your gut microbiome; this knowledge will only get more precise in the future. For example, looking at your gut microbiome can determine whether you are likely to develop Parkinson's syndrome for example. It's also possible to identify microbiome compositions that are more commonly found in people with certain conditions such as autism.

We are looking at this future: one where our enhanced understanding of the gut could revolutionize how we predict, diagnose, and most importantly, treat diseases. We already use the identification of certain genes to assess and determine this, but using the gut microbiome could offer even more specific results. It may at some point be able to predict how an individual will respond to a particular diet based on their gut microbiome. This is already being used in my practice, and future advancements will help us personalize our approach even more.

Recently, the ACS Science Journal published a study looking at a specific metabolic compound called triterpenoid, an antioxidant found to be very low in individuals with Parkinson's disease. It could also be indicative that an individual is at risk of developing Parkinson's disease later in life. Interestingly, this metabolite is found in foods like apples, spinach, and tomatoes.

It's thought that triterpenoid is neuroprotective because it reduces the oxidative stress that is released by free radicals in the brain. The study found a correlation between having low levels of triterpenoids and increased oxidative stress—which made the person more vulnerable to Parkinson's disease. Using this method increases the accuracy with which doctors can predict whether someone is likely to develop Parkinson's disease, providing a 96% accuracy.

Of course, predicting is useful, but it only goes so far—and the link with triterpenoids could actually offer us potential ways of preventing the disease. If part of the issue lies in the microbiome, we may be able to manipulate and change that, reducing someone's risk of developing a specific condition in the future.

The Potential of Fecal Microbiota Transplantation

There's another fascinating area in which learning about the power of the gut microbiome can help us unlock some incredible new healing potential for the world of medicine—a process called fecal microbiota transplantation (FMT). This involves transferring the fecal matter from a healthy individual into the gut of an individual who is unwell to introduce and establish healthy gut microbiota that may be deficient in the unhealthy gut. That might sound pretty incredible and unorthodox, but it has already been proven as a successful method of treating certain conditions, including recurrent Clostridium difficile infections—a serious condition that can be resistant to other treatments.

There's a lot of interest in exploring the potential this treatment has for other gut disorders, including IBS and IBD. At the moment, it's in its early stages, and there are several challenges, including standardizing protocols, identifying the traits of an optimal donor, and ensuring patient safety. However, as we better understand the gut and the interactions of the bacteria there, we may see FMT becoming a common approach for treating a variety of conditions.

The Importance of Continued Exploration for a Healthier Future

Although we have discussed reams of incredible information about how the gut affects almost every aspect of your health and wellness, it's important to note that we're really only scratching the surface of the gut microbiome and its phenomenal potential. In the future, we may see things like personalized probiotics, microbiome-based diagnostic tools, and microbiota-targeted therapies. As we go deeper into the microbial world and start to unlock the wonders within, our abilities to heal will grow exponentially. Committing to research and innovation could see us holding the keys to solving many of today's most harmful medical issues.

The Dangers of Using the Gut as a Bioweapon

However, all of these wonderful new ideas also come with a significant negative side, and this brings us to a much more controversial take on our new understanding of the microbiome. As we learn how to manipulate it so that we can cure diseases, we also have to recognize that there's a risk of this new understanding being utilized as a bioweapon.

This is because we can, theoretically, engineer dysbiosis—that condition we've discussed that leaves you far more vulnerable to diseases. We now know that giving people certain substances or different kinds of foods will change their microbiome, impacting their health and wellness. We can even modify and damage certain DNA, which causes problems for the microorganisms in the gut, thereby affecting the immune system.

For example, let's look at the COVID-19 vaccine. We know that having high levels of Bifidobacterium helps to protect you against severe COVID-19 infections, and people with adequate levels tend to experience much milder symptoms. Furthermore, we've seen that COVID-19 depleted Bifidobacterium in the gut, so the virus played havoc with our microbiome. Some studies have shown that the vaccine also depletes Bifidobacterium. It's unknown whether the depletion is caused by the COVID-19 nanoparticles contained within the vaccine or whether there is another reason. Once we understand that the gut microbiome can be disrupted and that this fundamentally affects how we respond to diseases, we need to consider the risks and benefits. It could revolutionize our ability to treat certain diseases, but it also carries some serious risks that deserve careful consideration as we continue moving forward. It's important for us to be aware of these risks, to account for them, and to encourage ethical practices in all ways. We have a tool that may offer us unprecedented power to heal, and we need to ensure we are using it as such.

Regardless of these advances, our gut is capable of being a potent "medicine cabinet" if we nourish it with what it needs for survival.

Things to Remember

- **Technological advancements** like NGS, and AI are propelling gut health research into a new era of personalized medicine.
- **Personalized nutrition based on microbiome data** has the potential to revolutionize dietary interventions.
- **Fecal microbiota transplantation** shows great promise for treating gut-related disorders, despite its challenges.
- **Continued research and exploration** into the complexities of the gut microbiome are critical for unlocking its full potential for health and well-being.
- **Stay informed about the latest developments** in gut health research and consider how they might apply to your personal health journey.
- **Discuss potentially integrating new diagnostic tools or therapeutic approaches** with your healthcare provider, including personalized nutrition or FMT.

- **Advocate for increased funding and support** for gut health research, given its potential to revolutionize our understanding of health and disease.

Glossary

Term	Definition
Acetylcholine	*Neurotransmitter involved in muscle activation and memory*
Adaptive immune system	*Body's defense mechanism that adapts to specific pathogens*
Antioxidants	*Compounds that prevent oxidative damage to cells*
Apoptosis	*Programmed cell death*
Aspartame	*Artificial sweetener*
Autophagy	*Cellular process of recycling damaged components*
B cells	*White blood cells producing antibodies*
Biofilm	*Community of microorganisms adhering to surfaces*
BPAs	*Chemicals used in making plastics*
CFU count	*Measurement of viable bacterial or fungal cells*
Cytokines	*Signaling proteins in immune responses*
Dopamine	*Neurotransmitter associated with pleasure and reward*
Dysbiosis	*Imbalance of gut microbiota*

Term	Definition
Fluoride	Mineral used to prevent tooth decay
Free radicals	Unstable molecules causing cellular damage
GABA	Neurotransmitter that inhibits nervous activity
Ghrelin	Hormone that stimulates appetite
Gluconeogenesis	Production of glucose from noncarbohydrate sources
Glycogenolysis	Breakdown of glycogen to glucose
Glyphosate	Herbicide used to kill weeds
Inflammatory bowel disease (IBD)	Chronic inflammation of the digestive tract
Innate immune system	Body's initial defense mechanism against pathogens
Interleukins	Cytokines that regulate immune responses
Inulin	Prebiotic fiber promoting gut health
Iodine	Mineral essential for thyroid function
Irritable bowel syndrome (IBS)	Disorder affecting bowel function
Ketosis	Metabolic state of burning fat for energy
Leaky gut	Increased intestinal permeability
Leptin	Hormone regulating hunger and fat storage
Lignans	Plant compounds with antioxidant properties
Lipopolysaccharides (LPS)	Molecules found in the outer membrane of certain bacteria

Term	Definition
Methylation	*Chemical process affecting gene expression*
Microbe	*Microscopic organism like bacteria or fungi*
Microbiome	*Community of microorganisms living in a specific environment*
MTHFR gene	*Gene involved in folate metabolism*
Neurotransmitters	*Chemicals transmitting signals in the nervous system*
Postbiotics	*Metabolic byproducts of probiotics*
Prebiotics	*Substances promoting the growth of beneficial bacteria*
Probiotics	*Live beneficial bacteria for gut health*
Psychobiotics	*Probiotics affecting mental health*
Red number 40	*Synthetic food dye*
Seed oils	*Oils extracted from seeds*
Serotonin	*Neurotransmitter regulating mood and digestion*
Short-chain fatty acids	*Fatty acids produced by gut bacteria*
Sucralose	*Artificial sweetener*
Synbiotics	*Combination of prebiotics and probiotics*
T cells	*White blood cells crucial for immune response*

References

Alcock, J., Maley, C. C., & Aktipis, C. A. (2014). Is eating behavior manipulated by the gastrointestinal microbiota? Evolutionary pressures and potential mechanisms. *BioEssays* 36(10), 940–949.

Ames, B. N., Grant, W. B., & Willett, W.C. (2021 Feb) Does the high prevalence of vitamin D deficiency in African Americans contribute to health disparities? *Nutrients* 13(2), 499, doi: 10.3390/nu13020499.

Arboleya, S., Watkins, C., Stanton, C., Ross, R. P.(2016). Gut bifidobacteria populations in human health and aging. *Frontiers in Microbiology* 7, 1204, doi: 10.3389/fmicb.2016.01204.

Azad, M. B., Bridgman, S. L., Becker, A. B., & Kozyrskyj, A. L. (2014). Infant antibiotic exposure and the development of childhood overweight and central adiposity. *International Journal of Obesity* 38(10), 1290–1298.

Belkaid, Y., & Harrison, O. J. (2017). Homeostatic immunity and the microbiota. *Immunity* 46(4), 562–576.

Benedict, C., Vogel, H., Jonas, W., Woting, A., Blaut, M., Schürmann, A., & Cedernaes, J. (2016). Gut microbiota and glucometabolic alterations in response to recurrent partial sleep deprivation in normal-weight young individuals. *Molecular Metabolism* 5(12), 1175–1186.

Besedovsky, L., Lange, T., & Haack, M. (2019). The sleep-immune crosstalk in health and disease. *Physiological Reviews*, 99(3), 1325–1380.

Besedovsky, L., Lange, T., & Haack, M. (2019). The sleep-immune crosstalk in health and disease. *Physiological Reviews* 99(3), 1325–1380.

Besedovsky, L., Lange, T., & Haack, M. (2019). The sleep-immune crosstalk in health and disease. *Physiological Reviews* 99(3), 1325–1380.

References

Bishara, C. (2020). Could certain strains of gut bacteria play a role in the prevention and potential treatment of COVID-19 infections? *American Journal of Translational Medicine* 4(2), 75–94. Retrieved from https://ajtm.journals.publicknowledgeproject.org/index.php/ajtm/article/view/615 (accessed on April 18, 2024).

Bonaz, B., Bazin, T., & Pellissier, S. (2018). The microbiota-gut-brain axis: a pathway involving the vagus nerve. *Frontiers in Neuroscience* 12, https://doi.org/10.3389/fnins.2018.00049.

Bowe, W., Patel, N. B., & Logan, A. C. (2014). Acne vulgaris, probiotics and the gut-brain-skin axis: from anecdote to translational medicine. *Beneficial Microbes* 5(2), 185–199.

Bruhn, J. G., & Wolf, S. (1979). *Roseto Revisited: The Story of an Italian-American Community's Extraordinary Longevity.* Harper & Row.

Bunyavanich, S., & Schadt, E. E. (2015). Systems biology of asthma and allergic diseases: a multiscale approach. *The Journal of Allergy and Clinical Immunology* 135(1), 31–42.

Cantorna, M. T., McDaniel, K., Bora, S., Chen, J., & James, J. (2020). Vitamin D, immune regulation, the microbiota, and inflammatory bowel disease. *Experimental Biology and Medicine* 245(1), 4–10.

Carlson, A. L., Xia, K., Azcarate-Peril, M. A., Goldman, B. D., Ahn, M., Styner, M. A., ... & Knickmeyer, R. C. (2018). Infant gut microbiome associated with cognitive development. *Biological Psychiatry* 83(2), 148–159.

Clarke, S. F., Murphy, E. F., O'Sullivan, O., Lucey, A. J., Humphreys, M., Hogan, A., Hayes, P., O'Reilly, M., Jeffery, I. B., Wood-Martin, R., Kerins, D. M., Quigley, E., Ross, R. P., O'Toole, P. W., Molloy, M. G., Falvey, E., Shanahan, F., & Cotter, P. D. (2014). Impact of exercise and dietary extremes on gut microbial diversity. *Gut* 63(12), 1913–1920, https://doi.org/10.1136/gutjnl-2013-306541.

Costa, R. J. S., Snipe, R., Kitic, C. M., & Gibson, P. R. (2019). Systematic review: exercise-induced gastrointestinal syndrome—implications for health and intestinal disease. *Alimentary Pharmacology & Therapeutics* 50(3), 246–265.

Dao, M. C., Everard, A., Aron-Wisnewsky, J., Sokolovska, N., Prifti, E., Verger, E. O., ... & Le Chatelier, E. (2016). Akkermansia muciniphila and improved metabolic health during a dietary intervention in obesity: relationship with gut microbiome richness and ecology. *Gut* 65(3), 426–436.

Dinan, T. G., Stilling, R. M., Stanton, C., & Cryan, J. F. (2015). How gut microbes influence human behavior: a collective unconsciousness. *Journal of Psychiatric Research*, 63, 1–9, https://doi.org/10.1016/j.jpsychires.2015.02.021.

Erny, D., Hrabě de Angelis, A. L., Jaitin, D., Wieghofer, P., Staszewski, O., David, E., ... & Keren-Shaul, H. (2015). Host microbiota constantly control maturation and function of microglia in the CNS. *Nature Neuroscience* 18(7), 965–977.

Fasano, A. (2012). Leaky gut and autoimmune diseases. *Clinical Reviews in Allergy & Immunology* 42(1), 71–78.

Fehr, K., Moossavi, S., Sbihi, H., Boutin, R. C.T., Bode, L., Robertson, B., Yonemitsu, C., J. Field, C. J., Becker, A. B., Mandhane, P. J., Sears, M. R., Khafipour, E., Moraes, T. J., Subbarao, P., Finlay, B. B., Turvey, S. E., Meghan, B. A. (2020). Breastmilk feeding practices are associated with the co-occurrence of bacteria in mothers' milk and the infant gut: the CHILD Cohort Study. *Cell Host & Microbe* 28(2), 285–297.

Foster, J. A., Rinaman, L., & Cryan, J. F. (2017). Stress & the gut-brain axis: regulation by the microbiome. *Neurobiology of Stress* 7, 124–136.

Fung, T. C., Olson, C. A., & Hsiao, E. Y. (2017). Interactions between the microbiota, immune and nervous systems in health and disease. *Nature Neuroscience* 20(2), 145–155.

Gabel, K., Hoddy, K. K., Haggerty, N., Song, J., Kroeger, C. M., Trepanowski, J. F., ... & Varady, K. A. (2018). Effects of 8-hour time restricted feeding on body weight and metabolic disease risk factors in obese adults: a pilot study. *Nutrition and Healthy Aging* 4(4), 345–353.

Gareau, M. G., Wine, E., Rodrigues, D. M., Cho, J. H., Whary, M. T., Philpott, D. J., ... & Sherman, P. M. (2011). Bacterial infection causes stress-induced memory dysfunction in mice. *Gut* 60(3), 307–317.

References

Gibson, G. R., Hutkins, R., Sanders, M. E., Prescott, S. L., Reimer, R. A., Salminen, S. J., Scott, K., Stanton, C., Swanson, K. S., Cani, P. D., Verbeke, K., & Reid, G. (2017). Expert consensus document: The International Scientific Association for Probiotics and Prebiotics (ISAPP) consensus statement on the definition and scope of prebiotics. *Nature Reviews Gastroenterology & Hepatology* 14(8), 491–502.

Goldman, B. (2021). *Stanford study ties milder covid-19 symptoms to prior run-ins with other coronaviruses*. News Center, https://med.stanford.edu/news/all-news/2021/07/stanford-study-ties-milder-covid-19-symptoms-to-prior-run-ins-wi.html (accessed on April 18, 2024).

Hao, Q., Dong, B. R., & Wu, T. (2015). Probiotics for preventing acute upper respiratory tract infections. *Cochrane Database of Systematic Reviews* 2, CD006895.

Hazan, S., Dave, S., Barrows, B. D. O., Borody, T. J. (2022). Messenger RNA SARS-CoV-2 vaccines affect the gut microbiome. *The American Journal of Gastroenterology* 117(10S), e162, doi: 10.14309/01.ajg.0000857548.07509.09.

Hazan, S., Dave, S., Barrows, B. D. O., Borody, T. J. (2022). Persistent damage to the gut microbiome following messenger RNA SARS-CoV-2 vaccine. *The American Journal of Gastroenterology* 117(10S), e1429–e1430, doi: 10.14309/01.ajg.0000865036.78992.16.

Hill, C., Guarner, F., Reid, G., Gibson, G. R., Merenstein, D. J., Pot, B., ... & Calder, P. C. (2014). Expert consensus document: The International Scientific Association for Probiotics and Prebiotics consensus statement on the scope and appropriate use of the term probiotic. *Nature Reviews Gastroenterology & Hepatology* 11(8), 506–514.

Hill, C., Guarner, F., Reid, G., Gibson, G. R., Merenstein, D. J., Pot, B., Morelli, L., Canani, R. B., Flint, H. J., Salminen, S., Calder, P. C., & Sanders, M. E. (2014). The International Scientific Association for Probiotics and Prebiotics consensus statement on the scope and appropriate use of the term probiotic. *Nature Reviews Gastroenterology & Hepatology* 11(8), 506–514.

Holick, M. F. (2017). The vitamin D deficiency pandemic: approaches for diagnosis, treatment and prevention. *Reviews in Endocrine and Metabolic Disorders* 18(2), 153–165.

Holscher, H. D. (2017). Dietary fiber and prebiotics and the gastrointestinal microbiota. *Gut Microbes* 8(2), 172–184.

https://badgut.org/information-centre/a-z-digestive-topics/brain-gut-connection-and-ibs/ (accessed on May 16, 2024).

https://www.consumerreports.org/health/food-safety/smarter-should-you-wash-produce-with-baking-soda-a6385579987/ (accessed on May 16, 2024).

https://www.cureus.com/articles/154753-effectiveness-of-osteopathic-manipulative-treatment-in-treating-symptoms-of-irritable-bowel-syndrome-a-literature-review#!/ (accessed on May 16, 2024).

https://www.frontiersin.org/journals/microbiology/articles/10.3389/fmicb.2016.01204/full#:~:text=In%20a%20European%20population%2C%20the,(Table%201)%2C%20B (accessed on May 16, 2024).

https://www.nature.com/articles/s41598-023-37738-1 (accessed on May 16, 2024).

https://www.ncbi.nlm.nih.gov/pmc/articles/PMC6731443/ (accessed on May 16, 2024).

https://www.sciencedirect.com/science/article/abs/pii/S0882401020300395 (accessed on May 16, 2024).

https://www.telegraph.co.uk/science/2019/05/20/life-easier-humans-hunted-gathered-food-cambridge-university/ (accessed on May 16, 2024).

Human Microbiome Project Consortium. (2012). Structure, function and diversity of the healthy human microbiome. *Nature* 486(7402), 207–214.

Human Microbiome Project Consortium. (2012). Structure, function and diversity of the healthy human microbiome. *Nature* 486(7402), 207–214.

Hunter S, Flaten E, Petersen C, Gervain J, Werker JF, Trainor LJ, et al. (2023) Babies, bugs and brains: how the early microbiome associates with infant brain and behavior development. *PLoS One* 18(8): e0288689, https://doi.org/10.1371/journal.pone.0288689.

Isomura, E. T., Suna, S., Kurakami, H. et al. (2023). Not brushing teeth at night may increase the risk of cardiovascular disease. *Scientific Reports* 13, 10467, doi: https://doi.org/10.1038/s41598-023-37738-1.

References

Kahlon, M. K., Aksan, N., Aubrey, R., et al. (2021). Effect of layperson-delivered, empathy-focused program of telephone calls on loneliness, depression, and anxiety among adults during the COVID-19 pandemic: a randomized clinical trial. *JAMA Psychiatry* 78(6), 616–622, doi:10.1001/jamapsychiatry.2021.0113.

Karl, J. P., Margolis, L. M., Madslien, E. H., Murphy, N. E., Castellani, J. W., Gundersen, Y., ... & Pasiakos, S. M. (2018). Changes in intestinal microbiota composition and metabolism coincide with increased intestinal permeability in young adults under prolonged physiological stress. *American Journal of Physiology - Gastrointestinal and Liver Physiology* 314(6), G559–G571.

Kelly, J. R., Borre, Y., O' Brien, C., Patterson, E., El Aidy, S., Deane, J., Kennedy, P. J., Beers, S., Scott, K., Moloney, G., Hoban, A. E., Scott, L., Fitzgerald, P., Ross, P., Stanton, C., Clarke, G., Cryan, J. F., & Dinan, T. G. (2016). Depression-linked gut microbiota induces neurobehavioural changes in rats. *Journal of Psychiatric Research* 82, 109–118, https://doi.org/10.1016/j.jpsychires.2016.07.019.

Khoruts, A., Rank, K. M., Newman, K. M., Viskocil, K., Vaughn, B. P., Hamilton, M. J., & Sadowsky, M. J. (2020). Inflammatory bowel disease affects the outcome of fecal microbiota transplantation for recurrent Clostridium difficile infection. *Clinical Gastroenterology and Hepatology* 15(8), 1154–1159.

Kong, H. H., Oh, J., Deming, C., Conlan, S., Grice, E. A., Beatson, M. A., ... & Nomicos, E. (2017). Temporal shifts in the skin microbiome associated with disease flares and treatment in children with atopic dermatitis. *Genome Research* 22(5), 850–859.

Konturek, P. C., Brzozowski, T., & Konturek, S. J. (2011). Gut and stress: pathophysiology, clinical consequences, diagnostic approach, and treatment options. *Journal of Physiology and Pharmacology: An Official Journal of the Polish Physiological Society* 62(6), 591–599.

Korem, T., Zeevi, D., Zmora, N., Weissbrod, O., Bar, N., Lotan-Pompan, M., ... & Suez, J. (2017). Bread affects clinical parameters and induces gut microbiome-associated personal glycemic responses. *Cell Metabolism* 25(6), 1243–1253.

Kostic, A. D., Chun, E., Robertson, L., Glickman, J. N., Gallini, C. A., Michaud, M., ... & Garrett, W. S. (2013). Fusobacterium nucleatum potentiates intestinal tumorigenesis and modulates the tumor-immune microenvironment. *Cell Host & Microbe* 14(2), 207–215.

Kuznia, S., Zhu, A., Akutsu, T., Buring, J. E., Camargo, C. A., Jr, Cook, N. R., Chen, L. J., Cheng, T. D., Hantunen, S., Lee, I. M., Manson, J. E., Neale, R. E., Scragg, R., Shadyab, A. H., Sha, S., Sluyter, J., Tuomainen, T. P., Urashima, M., Virtanen, J. K., Voutilainen, A., Wactawski-Wende, J., Waterhouse, M., Brenner, H., & Schöttker, B. (2023 Jun) Efficacy of vitamin D3 supplementation on cancer mortality: systematic review and individual patient data meta-analysis of randomised controlled trials. *Ageing Research Reviews* 87, 101923, doi: 10.1016/j.arr.2023.101923, Epub Mar 31, 2023.

Kwon, Y. H., Banskota, S., Wang, H., Rossi, L., Grondin, J. A., Syed, S. A., Yousefi, Y., Schertzer, J. D., Morrison, K. M., Wade, M. G., Holloway, A. C., Surette, M. G., Steinberg, G. R., & Khan, W. I. (2022). Chronic exposure to synthetic food colorant Allura Red AC promotes susceptibility to experimental colitis via intestinal serotonin in mice. *Nature Communications* 13(1), doi: 10.1038/s41467-022-35309-y.

Le Chatelier, E., Nielsen, T., Qin, J., Prifti, E., Hildebrand, F., Falony, G., ... & Sunagawa, S. (2013). Richness of human gut microbiome correlates with metabolic markers. *Nature* 500(7464), 541–546.

LeBlanc, J. G., Milani, C., de Giori, G. S., Sesma, F., van Sinderen, D., & Ventura, M. (2013). Bacteria as vitamin suppliers to their host: a gut microbiota perspective. *Current Opinion in Biotechnology* 24(2), 160–168.

Levy, L. M., & Degnan, A. J. (2013). GABA-based evaluation of neurologic conditions: MR spectroscopy. *AJNR: American Journal of Neuroradiology* 34(2), 259–265.

Ley, R. E., Turnbaugh, P. J., Klein, S., & Gordon, J. I. (2006). Microbial ecology: human gut microbes associated with obesity. *Nature* 444(7122), 1022–1023.

Ley, R. E., Turnbaugh, P. J., Klein, S., & Gordon, J. I. (2006). Microbial ecology: human gut microbes associated with obesity. *Nature* 444, 1022–1023.

Licht, T. R., Hansen, M., Bergström, A., & Poulsen, M. (2018). Effects of apples and specific apple components on the cecal environment of conventional rats: role of apple pectin. *BMC Microbiology* 10(1), 13.

Liu, Z., Dai, X., Zhang, H., Shi, R., Hui, Y., Jin, X., ... & Liu, C. (2017). Gut microbiota mediates intermittent-fasting alleviation of diabetes-induced cognitive impairment. *Nature Communications* 11(1), 1–12.

Longo, V. D., & Mattson, M. P. (2014). Fasting: molecular mechanisms and clinical applications. *Cell Metabolism* 19(2), 181–192.

Mailing, L. J., Allen, J. M., Buford, T. W., Fields, C. J., & Woods, J. A. (2019). Exercise and the gut microbiome: a review of the evidence, potential mechanisms, and implications for human health. *Exercise and Sport Sciences Reviews* 47(2), 75.

Mattson, M. P., Longo, V. D., & Harvie, M. (2017). Impact of intermittent fasting on health and disease processes. *Ageing Research Reviews* 39, 46–58.

Mayer, E. A., Knight, R., Mazmanian, S. K., Cryan, J. F., & Tillisch, K. (2014). Gut microbes and the brain: paradigm shift in neuroscience. *Journal of Neuroscience* 34(46), 15490–15496.

Mika, A., Van Treuren, W., González, A., Herrera, J. J., Knight, R., & Fleshner, M. (2015). Impact of exercise on gut microbial composition and lean mass: comparison between juvenile and adult male F344 rats. *PLoS One* 10(5), e0125889, https://doi.org/10.1371/journal.pone.0125889.

Monda, V., Villano, I., Messina, A., Valenzano, A., Esposito, T., Moscatelli, F., ... & Messina, G. (2017). Exercise modifies the gut microbiota with positive health effects. *Oxidative Medicine and Cellular Longevity* 2017.

Mutlu, E. A., Comba, I. Y., Cho, T., Engen, P. A., Yazıcı, C., Soberanes, S., ... & Budinger, G. R. (2018). Inhalational exposure to particulate matter air pollution alters the composition of the gut microbiome. *Environmental Pollution*, 240, 817–830.

Olguín, H. J., Guzmán, D. C., García, E. H., & Mejía, G. B. (2016). The role of dopamine and its dysfunction as a consequence of oxidative stress. *Oxidative Medicine and Cellular Longevity* 2016, 9730467.

Palmnäs, M. S. A., Cowan, T. E., Bomhof, M. R., Su, J., Reimer, R. A., Vogel, H. J., Hittel, D. S., & Shearer, J. (2014). Low-dose aspartame consumption differentially affects gut microbiota-host metabolic interactions in the diet-induced obese rat. *PLoS One* 9(10), e109841.

Pandey, K. R., Naik, S. R., & Vakil, B. V. (2015). Probiotics, prebiotics and synbiotics - a review. *Journal of Food Science and Technology* 52(12), 7577–7587.

Parodi, A., Paolino, S., Greco, A., Drago, F., Mansi, C., Rebora, A., ... & Savarino, V. (2008). Small intestinal bacterial overgrowth in rosacea: clinical effectiveness of its eradication. *Clinical Gastroenterology and Hepatology* 6(7), 759–764.

Patti, G. J., Yanes, O., & Siuzdak, G. (2012). Innovation: metabolomics: the apogee of the omics trilogy. *Nature Reviews Molecular Cell Biology* 13(4), 263–269.

Picciotto, M. R., Higley, M. J., & Mineur, Y. S. (2012). Acetylcholine as a neuromodulator: cholinergic signaling shapes nervous system function and behavior. *Neuron* 76(1), 116–129.

Proal, A. D., & Marshall, T. G. (2018). Myalgic encephalomyelitis/chronic fatigue syndrome in the era of the human microbiome: persistent pathogens drive chronic symptoms by interfering with host metabolism, gene expression, and immunity. *Frontiers in Pediatrics* 6, 373.

Qin, J., Li, Y., Cai, Z., Li, S., Zhu, J., Zhang, F., ... & Wang, J. (2012). A metagenome-wide association study of gut microbiota in type 2 diabetes. *Nature* 490(7418), 55–60.

Rappaport, J. (2017). Changes in dietary iodine explains increasing incidence of breast cancer with distant involvement in young women. *Journal of Cancer* 8(2), 174–177, doi: 10.7150/jca.17835.

Remely, M., Hippe, B., Geretschlaeger, I., Stegmayer, S., Hoefinger, I., & Haslberger, A. (2015). Increased gut microbiota diversity and abundance of Faecalibacterium prausnitzii and Akkermansia after fasting: a pilot study. *Wiener Klinische Wochenschrift* 127(9–10), 394–398.

Rezaie, A., Buresi, M., Lembo, A., Lin, H., McCallum, R., Rao, S., ... & Pimentel, M. (2017). Hydrogen and methane-based breath testing in gastrointestinal disorders: The North American Consensus. *The American Journal of Gastroenterology* 112(5), 775–784.

Ríos-Covián, D., Ruas-Madiedo, P., Margolles, A., Gueimonde, M., de Los Reyes-Gavilán, C. G., & Salazar, N. (2016). Intestinal short-chain fatty acids and their link with diet and human health. *Frontiers in Microbiology* 7, 185.

Salem, I., Ramser, A., Isham, N., & Ghannoum, M. A. (2018). The gut microbiome as a major regulator of the gut-skin axis. *Frontiers in Microbiology* 9, 1459.

Samavat H, Kurzer MS. Estrogen metabolism and breast cancer. (2015). *Cancer Letters* 356(2 Pt A), 231–243, doi: 10.1016/j.canlet.2014.04.018.

Sánchez, B., Delgado, S., Blanco-Míguez, A., Lourenço, A., Gueimonde, M., & Margolles, A. (2017). Probiotics, gut microbiota, and their influence on host health and disease. *Molecular Nutrition & Food Research* 61(1), 1600240.

Sarkar, A., Lehto, S. M., Harty, S., Dinan, T. G., Cryan, J. F., & Burnet, P. W. (2018). Psychobiotics and the manipulation of bacteria–gut–brain signals. *Trends in Neurosciences* 39(11), 763–781.

Sartor, R. B. (2008). Microbial influences in inflammatory bowel diseases. *Gastroenterology* 134(2), 577–594.

Scher, J. U., Sczesnak, A., Longman, R. S., Segata, N., Ubeda, C., Bielski, C., ... & Abramson, S. B. (2013). Expansion of intestinal Prevotella copri correlates with enhanced susceptibility to arthritis. *Elife* 2, e01202.

Schiffman, S. S., Scholl, E. H., Furey, T. S., & Nagle, H. T. (2023). Toxicological and pharmacokinetic properties of sucralose-6-acetate and its parent sucralose: *in vitro* screening assays. *Journal of Toxicology and Environmental Health* Part B, 26(6), 307–341, doi: 10.1080/10937404.2023.2213903.

Schloss, P. D., & Westcott, S. L. (2019). Identifying and overcoming threats to reproducibility, replicability, robustness, and generalizability in microbiome research. *mBio* 10(3), e00525–19.

Schwiertz, A., Taras, D., Schäfer, K., Beijer, S., Bos, N. A., Donus, C., & Hardt, P. D. (2011). Microbiota and SCFA in lean and overweight healthy subjects. *Obesity* 18(1), 190–195.

Scott, K. P., Martin, J. C., Campbell, G., Mayer, C. D., & Flint, H. J. (2006). Whole-genome transcription profiling reveals genes up-regulated by growth on fucose in the human gut bacterium "Roseburia inulinivorans." *Journal of Bacteriology* 188(12), 4340–4349.

Simrén, M., Barbara, G., Flint, H. J., Spiegel, B. M., Spiller, R. C., Vanner, S., ... & Zoetendal, E. G. (2013). Intestinal microbiota in functional bowel disorders: a Rome foundation report. *Gut* 62(1), 159–176.

Slavin, J. (2013). Fiber and prebiotics: mechanisms and health benefits. *Nutrients* 5(4), 1417–1435.

Thaiss, C. A., Zeevi, D., Levy, M., Zilberman-Schapira, G., Suez, J., Tengeler, A. C., ... & Korem, T. (2014). Transkingdom control of microbiota diurnal oscillations promotes metabolic homeostasis. *Cell* 159(3), 514–529.

Tilg, H., & Moschen, A. R. (2014). Microbiota and diabetes: an evolving relationship. *Gut* 63(9), 1513–1521.

Turroni, F., Peano, C., Pass, D. A., Foroni, E., Severgnini, M., Claesson, M. J., Kerr, C., Hourihane, J., Murray, D., Fuligni, F., Gueimonde, M., Margolles, A., De Bellis, G., O'Toole, P. W., van Sinderen, D., Marchesi, J. R., & Ventura, M. (2012). Diversity of bifidobacteria within the infant gut microbiota. *PLoS One* 7(5), e36957.

van Sadelhoff, J. H. J., van der Aa, L. B., van Doorn, M. B. A., Staats, C. C., El Ghalbzouri, A., & Knulst, A. C. (2019). The role of the gut-skin axis in the pathogenesis of acne: a comprehensive review. *Journal of Dermatological Science* 95(1), 21–27.

Vighi, G., Marcucci, F., Sensi, L., Di Cara, G., & Frati, F. (2008). Allergy and the gastrointestinal system. *Clinical and Experimental Immunology* 153(Suppl 1), 3–6.

Waterhouse, M., Hope, B., Krause, L., Morrison, M., Protani, M. M., Zakrzewski, M., & Neale, R. E. (2019). Vitamin D and the gut microbiome: a systematic review of in vivo studies. *European Journal of Nutrition* 58(7), 2895–2910.

Wei, B., Yunhong, W., Tingting, Y., Jiarong, Z., & Junlong, L. (2022). Women rely on "gut feeling"? The neural pattern of gender difference in non-mathematic intuition. *Personality and Individual Differences* 196, 111720, https://doi.org/10.1016/j.paid.2022.111720.

Why mice are used in Animal Research. EARA. (n.d.). https://www.eara. eu/mice-and-animal-research#:~:text=Mice%20have%20short%20 lifespans%20(2,develop%20and%20study%20in%20humans (accessed on April 18, 2024).

Yang, T., Doherty, J., Zhao, B., Kinchla, A. J., Clark, J. M., & He, L. (2017). Effectiveness of commercial and homemade washing Agents in removing pesticide residues on and in apples. *Journal of Agricultural and Food Chemistry* 65(44), 9744–9752.

Young, S. N. (2007). How to increase serotonin in the human brain without drugs. *Journal of Psychiatry & Neuroscience* 32(6), 394–399.

Zeeuwen, P. L., Kleerebezem, M., Timmerman, H. M., & Schalkwijk, J. (2013). Microbiome and skin diseases. *Current Opinion in Allergy and Clinical Immunology* 13(5), 514–520.

Zeevi, D., Korem, T., Zmora, N., Israeli, D., Rothschild, D., Weinberger, A., ... & Suez, J. (2015). Personalized nutrition by prediction of glycemic responses. *Cell* 163(5), 1079–1094.

Zhang, Y. K., Zhang, Q., Wang, Y. L., Zhang, W. Y., Hu, H. Q., Wu, H. Y., Sheng, X. Z., Luo, K. J., Zhang, H., Wang, M., Huang, R., Wang, G. Y. (2021). A comparison study of age and colorectal cancer-related gut bacteria. *Frontiers in Cellular and Infection Microbiology* 11, 606490. doi: 10.3389/fcimb.2021.606490, https://www.ncbi.nlm.nih.gov/pmc/ articles/PMC8121496/ (accessed on April 18, 2024).

Zitvogel, L., Daillère, R., Roberti, M. P., Routy, B., & Kroemer, G. (2017). Anticancer effects of the microbiome and its products. *Nature Reviews Microbiology* 15(8), 465–478.

Acknowledgment

I want to thank Global Book Publishing for all their guidance in getting this book published.

I would also like to thank my colleagues in science, Dr. Blaize and Dr. Sidime, who co-authored the Covid study. The real beauty of medicine is the collaboration of doctors and scientists with different expertise, coming together to heal others.

About the Author

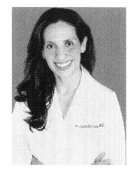

Christine Bishara, MD, is an integrative physician with a background in Internal Medicine. In her 20+ years of practicing medicine, she has come to the conclusion that the body is a powerful healer on its own, but sometimes needs some tools and direction to heal appropriately. The mind–body connection is a powerful one and is not utilized enough to help heal. By focusing on gut health, Dr. Bishara believes that this allows all body systems to work together in healing and strengthening the immune system. Dr. Bishara is also a pioneer in gut health and published the first peer-reviewed study linking COVID-19 severity to the deficiency of a vital, beneficial gut bacteria. The study also hypothesizes that this is the reason children did not become severely ill from COVID-19, due to the high presence of this beneficial bacteria in their gut.

Email: info@fromwithinmedical.com

Scan to Connect

Made in the USA
Middletown, DE
07 December 2024

66345804R00099